THE
SECRET ART
OF
SEAMM-JASANI

THE
SECRET ART
OF
SEAMM-JASANI

58 Movements for Eternal Youth from Ancient Tibet

ASANARO

Translated by Joice Buccarey C. and Benjamin B. Kelley
with drawings by Asanaro

JEREMY P. TARCHER / PUTNAM
A MEMBER OF PENGUIN GROUP (USA) INC. * NEW YORK

Most Tarcher/Putnam books are available at special quantity discounts for bulk purchase for sales promotions, premiums, fund-raising, and educational needs. Special books or book excerpts also can be created to fit specific needs. For details, write Penguin Group (USA) Inc. Special Markets, 375 Hudson Street, New York, NY 10014.

Jeremy P. Tarcher/Putnam
a member of
Penguin Group (USA) Inc.
375 Hudson Street
New York, NY 10014
www.penguin.com

Published simultaneously in Canada

Library of Congress Cataloging-in-Publication Data

Asanaro, date.
The secret art of Seamm-Jasani : 58 movements for eternal youth from ancient Tibet / by
Asanaro ; translated by Joice Buccarey C. and Benjamin B. Kelley ;
with drawings by Asanaro.
p.   cm.
ISBN 1-58542-241-X
1. Self-care, Health—China—Tibet.   2. Medicine, Tibetan.
3. Exercise—China—Tibet.   I. Title.
RA776.95.A84   2003   2002044738
613'.0951'5—dc21

Printed in the United States of America
7   9   10   8   6

This book is printed on acid-free paper. ∞

Book design by Lovedog Studio

My most sincere energies and recognition

to my special students

Amlom and Ben,

whose hard work and patience

made this translation possible.

Asanaro

CONTENTS

THE
SECRET ART
OF
SEAMM-JASANI

by Asanaro
in the year of the Isebom

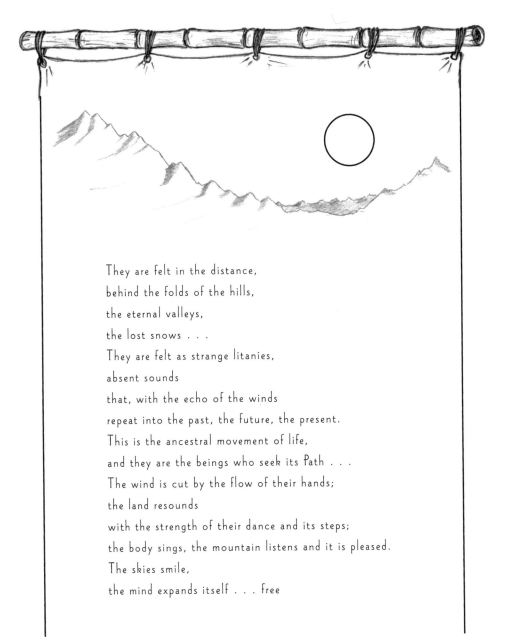

They are felt in the distance,
behind the folds of the hills,
the eternal valleys,
the lost snows . . .
They are felt as strange litanies,
absent sounds
that, with the echo of the winds
repeat into the past, the future, the present.
This is the ancestral movement of life,
and they are the beings who seek its Path . . .
The wind is cut by the flow of their hands;
the land resounds
with the strength of their dance and its steps;
the body sings, the mountain listens and it is pleased.
The skies smile,
the mind expands itself . . . free

INTRODUCTION

I T WAS JUST dawn . . . the morning cold fading away as the sun won one more day in its eternal movement. Step by step, all of the life in those solitary mountains crept back into its natural rhythm, flourishing again after the winter of night. Small birds began their morning flights as the apprentices of the Path finished the dawn's work. A delicate fog trickled through the hillsides and the valleys as if embracing them, blanketing them with an invisible, protective gown that dissipated slowly as the great star-sun shone its face over the summits. It was time to feed the necessary warmth to the body and mind, to begin once again the work of the day. The deep blue sky encouraged the enjoyment of their chores; the heat, as the sun grew up into the sky, was perfect for beginning the first movements of the body in the "Path of the Art."

. . .

The guide in charge of this group of apprentices had awoken long ago—it was rare to find him still asleep at this time. Everyone awaited anxiously the morning's new lesson: years ago they had been initiated into the Art of Awakening, the Art of Relaxation, the Art of Breathing, and the hermetic Osseous Art, reserved for so few. All deeply appreciated these teachings, one amongst them more so than the others.

"Perhaps," this restless apprentice wondered, "they being so few that know these secrets, perhaps one day its transmission and inheritance will be lost, one more treasure buried in time, no one left to give it life or vibrate with its teachings; an old dinosaur, survivor of an antediluvian era, it would be condemned and extinguished." In the middle of his thoughts the guide interrupted him.

"Suam Odaonai! The energy is strong and open today . . . why do you want to use it all up in doubt?" were the words that, with certainty, interrupted the thoughts that had taken possession of the student.

"I was thinking about the teachings . . ."

"Yes, I already know," was the answer.

"I am thinking of the future, and I dislike the thought that one day your Art may be lost, that no one else will be able to follow it properly or understand it completely."

"When you think, you doubt, instinctively, and that moves you away from the real answer. The Art has life in the mind and in the body of one who is willing to understand it, to practice it, and to follow it as a way of life. The Art that I transmit to you needs neither time nor followers, nor to shock ignorant masses that hear only what they wish, who read what has been censored and made comfortable to their mistaken lives, all full of concepts of ambition, jealousy, materialism, self-destruction, the devaluation of others and of themselves. Wisdom is not enlarged by numbers."

"The guide always has a very direct way of speaking; those who know him understand him," the apprentice thought. However, he asked anyway.

"But what do you mean by that . . . ?"

"It is very simple: every living being possesses an 'art' by which it understands life. This understanding, almost every time, is based on assumptions imposed upon it by a predetermined environment. The strong one dominates the weak one who follows the proposition of the stronger as to how he should exist; this is the reason people will follow paths that are not their own, as among humans, for example, drug use and alcoholism. The weak support the strong and in the end they all take the simplest road. There is no being that by its own nature believes in the self-destruction caused by drugs, alcoholism, or tobacco; these are habits imposed and given the appearance of normalcy. Think about this and remember what you have seen . . . the worst evil is that which has the appearance of good."

"But if they knew our Art they could improve many facets of that mistaken life," the apprentice answered.

"First, look at and value yourself. The Art is complicated: it needs discipline, perseverance, and, most important, a search and desire for perfection; for common people, it implies a prohibition, for they only have time to listen to negative things, to smoke, to make their own lives a misery, and to make the lives of others even worse, which is their favorite sport. Besides, it is much easier, much more comfortable, to follow the thoughts of others than to think for ourselves, to make the same mistakes as everyone else without overcoming our own, to think in the past and not in the present, to think about the future, just as you are doing right now, and not vibrating to the maximum in the present moment."

"You are completely right . . ."

"This is not about being right or wrong, it is about making clear that which we all know, which is the truth . . . But this is hard to accept."

"But, if people understood or if people wanted to understand more, they would really feel the difference of knowing this teaching; it would make their lives much richer . . ." added the student, which immediately brought a new answer.

"Yes . . . and that is not all. They would live forever . . ."

"But how! That is not possible!" answered the amazed apprentice. The guide just smiled to himself, paused for a second, and said:

"The important thing is not what is or is not possible. Those two ideas limit you. The important thing is that if you use your mind in a positive way everything can be possible."

"But can you really enlarge your life with the Art's movements?"

"Learn and you will find the answer by yourself: you know well, and you have seen this in practice, that every human mind has two different organs, or magnetic elements, that are highly sensitive, transmitting energy to the rest of the body while simultaneously making you emanate an electric field or aura that surrounds you completely; it is a shame, for these organs are numb, almost totally unused. Those who think in the external world find it very difficult to recognize that this latent energy exists in every living being; however, slowly they will realize it . . . this is something that is inevitable. Right now, their materialism does not allow them to go beyond where they are. When they see a rat they do not see a sensitive being, they see only one more object to experiment on; this thinking doesn't allow them to obtain the completely correct results that they seek. If they had in mind those two organs, they would realize that we are not just individualistic chemistry but an entire magnetic field. Think about this and you'll see that everything is movement, that everything is interdependent vibration, and that we are constantly emanating and receiving energy.

"When we learn the first movements and breathing forms we begin to break the cycle or routine that every being creates for itself. This routine creates certain static connections in the mind. It leaves ripples, or furrows as in a field, through which we must walk. Usually, people living in the cities wake up in the morning after a bad night and without having completely rested: their energy is weak and they begin their day with a cup of coffee to compensate the physical and internal fatigue that they carry. To make things even worse, they smoke a cigarette, trying to cover an already ugly thing with more garbage. The already weak energy that surrounds them weakens even more. When they go to work they meet different people, each one with a different and generally negative mood, each with their own, similarly depressed, energy. This collides with the energy of the person in our example, creating negative waves and weakening even more this force that surrounds him or her, penetrating it easily. Through expressions of dislike, hard or strong words, through pejorative or cold looks, this energy flows faster and enters directly into the interior of this already weak person. Imagine him, his energy field lowered, sleepless, with tobacco and other toxins in his body, in a cold, competitive environment where the people who surround him emanate their own negative energy; this poor person tenses his nervous system completely, top to bottom, and the flow of energy is interrupted as he takes in only the negative from his surroundings.

"Perhaps you will find this example a bit exaggerated," the guide continues, "but in its essence it happens to everyone. If you are not like this, not the way things actually are all over this world; if you are different, honest, and too positive, your expulsion is final!" the guide and the apprentice both smiled. "But, continuing with our earlier discussion . . . as the day goes by, the energy of our person weakens more and more with every encounter. Evening comes and, after accumulating all of this negative energy, his only desire will be to unload everything in any possible way: he will try with his family, yelling at his partner, gossiping about the neighbors, expressing his intolerance and prejudice. Imagine him, in this exact moment instinctively beginning all of these tremendous arguments in order to discharge his negative energy. . . . Obviously even this is not completely achieved and all that is really created is a heightened transmission of negative energy to everybody else, thus repeating this vicious cycle. If continually fighting with others isn't bad enough—and this is the worst part of it all—out of all of this, illness, discouragement, and premature aging are born."

By this time the sun had nicely warmed up, announcing a beautiful day, perfect for learning and for listening to words that nourish internal energy.

The apprentice asked, curiously, "But in what way does our Art change that cycle?"

"Keep quiet, listen, and learn," said the guide, half joking and half serious. "The Art is a cycle of movements, and well you have learned that every action brings a reaction. Because of this, if this person of whom we have spoken, under his constant strain of tension, discovered during his life our Arts and their secrets, even if superficially, he would find great relief from his real illness: the weakness of his magnetic organs, and from this, the terrible consequences to his mind, his body, and his defenses, both internal and aurical. He would leave behind the weaknesses that consume his inner energy and that, as part of a monotonous life, will cause him a painful or premature death. With the Art, life takes motion and follows its normal course, makes the one who learns it and takes it to heart flourish from the inside. Because of this every movement executed moves these magnetic organs as if they were an old rusty door that we patiently repair, lubricate, and finally move again . . . so they can open! Think, the function creates the organ, the movement recreates the inner mind so the magnetic fields work again, starting with simple mental-physical coordinations.

"Everyone walks, yet they do not think about walking; it is all subconscious. The same for sweeping, or for playing with a ball. . . . But could they walk, sweep with one hand, and play with a ball in the other, all at the same time? It would be difficult, and that is what our teaching is about in some way, because it forces us to unite different roads: mind, breath, imagination, movement, projection, all at the same time. A person could revive in himself the teachings of the ancestors for the Full Life, for Eternal Vitality. His magnetic or energy field, born in the organs that I mentioned before, would be strengthened now, powerful and brilliant. His 'aura,' if you wish to call it that, would grow. If this person were to learn to use his body and imagination in a positive way, he would see everything begin to improve around him. Now, when waking up in the morning he would be in a good mood. He would be completely rested and would begin the day happy, with a lucid mind and positive thoughts; his need for tobacco would decrease significantly within him, until it vanished unnoticed; his energy, now revitalized and solid, would be ready to face the day in a new way, with more calm and more strength. He would have to deal with negative people anyway, but their depressing energy would simply bounce off of him. In this way he could greatly reduce the 'internal nervous contraction' so disastrous for vitality. Thus he would come closer to Eternal Youth, Eternal Vitality, and the Great Inner Energy.

"Imagine that, from a certain point of view, these movements are like an electrical ground that all of us need. This ground discharges all of our negative energy and allows us to dedicate all of our strength, all of the time, to our own evolution. Otherwise it is as if we were in a boat with too much ballast, or in one that is constantly leaking: it will inevitably sink before its time, take too long to arrive, or simply remain stranded behind on the journey. This teaching brings with it health, stability, and the enlarging of Youth and Life, for it works as a bilge pump on our boat, removing our dead weight, so we can use all of our 'organic time' toward advance, self-healing, and inner recovery."

"Guide, someday I would like to write about this Art, so that people might get to know it and be helped by it," the apprentice said.

"If you were to do that, most people wouldn't understand it and they would be much more willing to criticize and destroy than to experience it, for people possess in general a very negative and depressed inner energy, which manifests itself spontaneously. Envy, gossip, and incomprehension rule everywhere: humankind is nowadays profoundly shocked and is like a sick person who is struggling to heal. Materialism uses them; prejudices and fear of difference dominates. People are still convalescents, the heirs of hundreds of years of much persecution, war, repression, and much, so very much fear and prejudice toward difference . . . all imposed by convenience. Recall the Great Universal Record, how wise and inquisitive people were misunderstood and persecuted in different epochs; you have the clear example of Socrates of Athens, infamously sentenced to death for 'corrupting the youth' and for 'not worshipping' the gods who were in fashion. This argument has been repeated too many times in the course of human history: ignorance, intolerance, and power are a terrible and dangerous combination. If we advance eight hundred years, you will see an earth unevolved, except that this time it is Hypatia of Alexandria, an astronomer and physicist known for her scientific and academic excellence, also the last custodian of the great library. Knowledge is a dangerous thing and those who rule see it as a risk; thus she was flayed by the ruling sect, simply for her desire to preserve ancient writings that collected sciences, arts, and technology: books that in a thousand years could have advanced the knowledge of all of humanity. You know well that the stupidity that reigned during that time permitted the domination of the minds of the masses, who went happily to the murder of Hypatia. She committed the two worst possible errors that she could have, had she wished to survive in such an obtuse, dark, and decadent world: first, to be a woman, and second, to protect knowledge. The worst thing of all is that this era of confusion has continued for a very long time; thus, twelve hundred years later, someone like Galileo Galilei was judged, tormented, and persecuted because he affirmed that the Earth revolved around the Sun. Ignorance nearly killed again, because this individual wanted to help others by lifting them out of mediocrity. . . . Humanity has suffered too much and that makes it dangerous, as a soldier who has been in too many wars, seen too many crimes. . . . He carries a terrible weight with him; in this same way the world carries a terrible weight on its back, and as long as it does not rid itself completely of this weight, science and wisdom should be well preserved and kept a secret, for otherwise they will be handled wrongfully, persecuted, and misunderstood."

"But, despite that, there would be some who would under-stand, who would value and enjoy our knowledge, and they would live a better life with great benefits . . ."

"There will always be people who value our Art, this is certain, or at least accept it without prejudice. For the rest of the people, those who are narrow-minded, those who condemned Socrates, who murdered Hypatia, or judged Galileo . . . for all of them, the Path of Eternal Youth will remain forever an Ancient and Millen-nial Secret Art, hermetic and mysterious, like it has had to be to this very day . . ."

At this moment it was time to begin the morning class. The guide stood up as they all gathered around him and went to a small esplanade that they had prepared for the occasion. It was a special place, a natural field of grass with a few stones moved to form a large circle that demarcated the place of teaching. Some branches that had fallen from trees had been carefully tied with dried grass into a strange symbol at the front of the circle. Once everything was prepared they made flowing gestures with their arms, a cere-monious greeting, and the guide began his dictation. He emitted a sonorous and rhythmic tone, like some methodical melody from a mountain dimension, or perhaps from another universe. The ap-prentices followed him in a strange dance; projections and steps moved united as their hands touched the air with flourishes, cut-ting it to produce soft sounds . . . the smooth movements of an old teaching. As a relic, lost in time and rediscovered, it took life in-side their bodies and inside each one of them. The mind ex-panded . . . free.

The apprentice was still restless, thinking one thing—if he wrote and transmitted what he had learned, how would he do it, what would be correct . . . how to explain, how to summarize and simplify so that everyone could understand. . . .

"Perhaps I would do it in eight stages . . ."

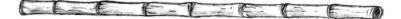

The Art of Discovering Eternal Youth

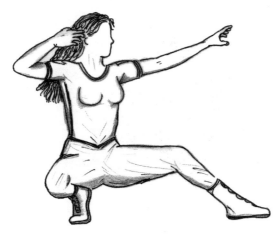

"The artist realizes himself in his work; the
mind realizes itself in life."

E VERY LIVING BEING'S existence is a constant struggle for life. Human beings, especially, wish for eternal life. This book is a small contribution toward the understanding of that search, not the useless pretension toward an endless existence but toward learning how to enjoy, to the utmost, what we have now.

The Art for Eternal Youth is a way of life: it is not so much about following a pattern of exercises as it is about vibrating, about preparing the mind toward the positive, the jovial, and the spontaneous smile. If a reader were to ask me what the formula for Eternal Youth is, I would answer that there is one that is inevitably the best, and its first *movement* is happiness.

When we speak of an Art, it makes us think of wisdom, of harmony, of universals, not of the cold theories of cells, their effective or ineffective oxidation, or the eternal genetic errors of reproduction. A correct scientific answer is unimportant; perhaps, if science will find it someday, it will be based in the depths of the mind, in the intrinsic beauty of things, in what is profound and delicate and so well kept in each one of us.

Many have already dedicated too many hours of study to the important aspects of food: trying to determine what to eat and what not to eat, transforming this into long lists of prohibitions, restrictions, combinations of acceptable and unacceptable foods. In the end this only bores us, as we don't know whether we get more depressed by not being able to follow all of the rules or by not being allowed to break any of them. This is the reason that I speak of an *Art* for Eternal Youth, and not a *technique* for Eternal Youth, as if it were some cold chemical formula. One can encounter people who have followed no special rules for living and have lived many years longer, and better, than those who have followed strict norms.

There are many people nowadays who talk a lot about genetics, which I think is sometimes more harmful than helpful to our lives; for if we limit ourselves to a preordained life span of a predetermined quality, we are predisposing ourselves to negativity and eliminating any possibility of evolving for ourselves. When we speak about the Art for Eternal Youth it means just that: to be an artist, to have a wholly positive mind, to be creative, to let your imagination run free and to follow your natural instinct toward spontaneity, as a child, without repressing yourself . . . letting your energy flow and remaining constantly in motion, so as not to stagnate and rot.

If I had to give advice as to the best exercises for maintaining a completely healthy body, I would have to ask, "Do you want a healthy, childlike, and powerful vision? Then watch the sun set, enjoy waves as they break on the seashore, follow with your eyes the beautiful lines of high mountains, enjoy the colors of flowers, and follow with curiosity your eyes' attraction to the darkness of the night, and the brightness of the stars." If someone were to ask me: "What shall I do to keep my hearing eternally sharp and young?" I would have to respond, "Listen to and enjoy the songs of birds, the whispering of the wind, the falling, beneficent rain, the crystalline sound of the river that runs unceasingly, as well as the constant motion of the waves." If the question was, "How are the perfect smell and the ideal taste of Eternal Youth cultivated?" I should say that there is nothing better than smelling the sweet scent of a field at dawn, tasting fruit just picked from a tree, drinking water fresh from a slope, smelling and tasting bread hot from the oven.

The idea behind *positive energy* is a capacity to enjoy things in a simple and transparent way; it is a way of playing, joking, and laughing as children, of being in a good mood and enjoying natural things, like walking barefoot on the beach or putting your feet in the mud without worrying about getting them dirty or wondering if there might be someone watching. This is why, in this book, I do not talk directly about food but about enjoying it. Even though moderation is always good advice, it really does not matter whether we eat meat or are strict vegetarians; what matters most is that we are happy carnivores or vegetarians (if you want to be young forever, enjoy everything). I still remember a trip I took to the mountains, where eating animal fat was like eating an appetizer, and butter soup like a glass of water. The air in those mountains, the walks we took, and the water from the slopes made heavy meals a necessity for every activity, and I am sure that if I had eaten this sort of food in the city, I would most likely have gone straight to the nearest hospital.

The Art for Eternal Youth begins with our actions, with our psychical-physical developments and the way that we handle our accumulated mental and physical load, all through a natural relationship with the food that we eat. We can have a perfect diet without being too strict, according to the area of the planet in which we live, and trying to keep in mind fruits, vegetables, cereals, and a lot of water. If you are one of those insistent people who enjoys following endless lists, and in fact feel some pleasure in doing so, I will give some advice (just advice) on healthy habits.

✱   Permanently abandon tobacco. This causes premature aging, brings on many different illnesses, and gives you septic-tank breath (please forgive my honesty). If this is not enough, smoking ruins your teeth, gives you cancer, damages your lungs, and fouls your blood, along with all of the logical consequences that accrue (high blood pressure, less food for your cells, a brain full of smoke, etcetera). Besides, have you thought about how much money you would save if you did not smoke? Or how much you will save, down the road, on doctors and medication?

✱   Absolutely avoid any and all varieties of drugs (unless, of course, it is medication prescribed by a responsible doctor— something totally different). Drugs are the worst enemy of health and of any desire to enlarge life, youth, or vitality. There are many beliefs and superstitions in eastern (and some western) religions that have given functionality as a "supernatural" stimulant to some toxic herbs (marijuana, etcetera), but this is some of the worst ignorance that could ever exist. If you want to see spectacular images from "beyond," you would be better off asking a "friend" to grab a baseball bat and hit you in the head, hard. I can guarantee that you would see squares, lights, even have a "divine revelation," all for free, and with far less consequence than comes with using drugs. If someone tells you with any conviction, even though they may sound reasonable, that drugs are good and that they will help you feel better, different, make you forget bad times, then that person is a complete lunatic and if you follow them you are even more of a lunatic. Drugs are the most harmful thing that you could possibly bring upon yourself and the people around you.

★ Be wise with alcohol. As everyone should know excess in alcohol kills, not only because an irresponsible drunk can be responsible for a serious accident, but also because it causes disease, known as cirrhosis. Besides, an alcoholic makes his relatives' lives miserable, and after a while they will take their revenge and make the alcoholic's life miserable, too. If you are going to drink, drink in moderation, mainly a good red wine drunk with food. The healthiest and most natural is handmade wine, which helps in the digestion of heavy meats and has the fashionably healthy attribute of being an antioxidant (they say that when people get older they start to "oxidize," which seems a bit metaphoric).

★ Avoid coffee and caffeinated tea. These drinks have well-known constituents that alter and directly attack your nervous system, and to live longer and better it is necessary to have very good nerves. You can replace these elements with herbal teas, or by toasting some apple and carrot skin in your oven. Once they are toasted put them in a teapot with boiling water, and there you have it: a natural tea free from toxins.

∗　Drink lots of water, several quarts a day if possible; this will keep your skin in excellent condition, will make your digestion easier, and will help to clean out your blood. Do not drink soda, as it is not good for anything, and the most popular ones taste like rotten syrup. Keep in mind that it is better to drink farther away from meals, and if you would like to drink something herbal I can recommend some healthier ones that are revitalizing and diuretic. Personally, they have really worked for me.

∗　Try not to eat meat every day. Meat is good, but it is not advisable to eat it too often, because it takes a lot of work to digest, which consumes a great amount of youth . . . I'm sorry . . . energy. Besides, it also increases the uric acid in your blood. It is better to eat meat once or twice a week, especially white meat cooked at home, of which it would be ideal (basically a synonym for impossible) for you to know the origin. Nowadays, the production of meat is quite dubious: chemicals, hormones, genetics, and animal foods made out of dead animals have produced only illnesses and horrible deformations. So, if you are a junk-food lover, don't be alarmed if one day you find a third eye in your forehead, or find hair where you didn't have it before, or see your breasts start to grow . . . don't worry, these are just the consequences of our modern era. It is said, as a joke, that, when we die, our bodies may turn into dust again, but our stomachs will stick around for a few hundred years because of all the chemicals and preservatives in the food we eat.

✴ Try to replace regular sugar with brown sugar, which is healthier. Honey is also a good substitute.

✴ Please, if you are older, don't spend the whole day talking about how old you are, what diseases you have, what new wrinkles have shown up in your face (this has nothing to do with food, but I needed to say it).

✴ Avoid too much salt.

✴ Eat lots of fruits, vegetables, and cereals.

✴ Try not to eat late at night, as it is better to go to sleep on an empty stomach (if you can do this, you have an advantage over me, because I am still one of those who can't quit eating before going to sleep).

✴ On the other hand, if you have one of modern society's diseases such as anorexia or bulimia, I can guarantee that you are not going to achieve anything aside from getting into the hospital or the cemetery. If you want to keep doing this, please be economical and get yourself some good health and life insurance.

*   Be sensible, follow a balanced path: food is something that is sacred, delicious, and necessary, and to see it as an enemy is just one more grand idiocy contributing to this competitive and conceited society.

*   *WHEN EATING: ENJOY IT!!!!!!!*

Now you have a whole lot of advice to have fun with. Later on in this book we will learn how to channel energy through the development of our Art, rather than through the foods we eat.

The forms that this book relays attempt to give a summary of how we can channel our daily accumulation of energy. We call this old science the *Art of Relaxation in Motion,* because while we are executing movements that help us burn calories, there is a simultaneous relaxation taking place, predisposing our minds toward a positive way of living. This is very important, for where a positive mind rules, there is no room for diseases.

When we begin to study this Art, we should also talk about it as Seamm-Jasani: "the Art for the Great Knowledge through Smooth Movements" (or as it was called in Sanskrit, "Alayavij-nana," although this also was not its own and original name).

The path of the Seamm-Jasani is not something recent; it comes from an ancient time, before Sanskrit, with roots beyond what we now call Tibet, or the East in general. Today, yoga from India and tai-chi from China are popularly known, but the Art that I describe preceeds them by thousands of years; it has been hermetically preserved by some families and is superior to those other techniques because of the docility of its movements, its dynamics, logic, elegance, and natural adaptation to the body without a need to adopt circus postures; while at the same time, the development of the movements is infinite and produces quick, concrete, and direct results. What I present in this book is only a humble summary of hundreds of physical-psychical coordinative and meditative techniques in this ancestral Art whose forgotten origins are in the lost valleys of what in its time was known as Peuyul, or Bod.

I am not trying to explain in this small book a complete wisdom that requires many years of study with a guide who is patient, wise, meticulous, and demanding in his teaching, as was the one to whom I was apprenticed. The roots of this Art, from which I have taken these techniques, will continue another ancient mystery that can only be transmitted orally and directly, not from a book. We are living in a time when it seems obligatory to reveal all secrets and wisdom, where everything must appear in the newspapers, libraries, or even on the Internet; but not all is this way, for there are still things that we must make an effort to learn: "nothing comes from nothing," an old saying goes, and real knowledge is only achieved by effort, values, and searching.

My intention in this book is to help the reader come closer to a science lost in time, which if not for this book would be impossible, or very improbable, for him or her to learn. It is also true that even if I wanted to (and this does not mean that I do), I could not explain "all" in this book. These writings are only an approach that, for everyone who makes an effort, will be easy to decipher. I have not used complicated names for the movements, as I prefer a simple and direct translation in good English, because the objective is that you work with your body and mind, not learn another language. Also, instead of elaborating a longer course, I have remained with what is most essential, simplest, and closest to everyone; after all, it would be neither correct nor responsible to describe technical elements that are impossible to learn if not taught directly, personally, with discipline and patience, as it was done in the old times: in three dimensions.

Don't worry, as you won't find complicated theorizations about "meridians," "parallels," and other references that I find more akin to descriptions on a map than to reality; I am not trying to be controversial, but I prefer the way that I learned: "Observe, experience, and feel everything by yourself." I do not make references to "chakras" either, because in my own life the only "chakras" that I have known are the places where delicious fruits and vegetables grow, watered by the rivers and fed by the sun of the southern hemisphere. (In [Chilean] Spanish, chakra means field.)

These writings attempt to summarize the most simple and universal techniques, across the high, medium, and low zones of the body, condensing the basic and fundamental movements so that anyone, whatever his or her age, can, with a little dedication, execute them without difficulty. Many of these exercises may be similar to others that you already know, because I have tried to make them universal, easy, and *practical*. It would be impossible to try to transmit the Seamm-Jasani and the other superior arts in a single book. This book is meant to be a vitamin to every conscientious reader, in order that he or she may practice, simply, techniques that have been zealously kept for thousands of years as a lifestyle, as natural self-medicine, and as a way to enlarge the energy of the body and the lucidity of the mind for as many years as possible.

What is most important is that, in just a couple of square yards, we can execute basic and entertaining movements that can help us in our lives on this planet. Think that any type of tension in you lowers your performance and your defenses, and therefore hampers your well-being and shortens your life. We are perfectly formed beings, with the capability for self-healing or self-destruction (which the practical tends to favor), and if we can begin to heal ourselves, we are one step closer to the source of eternal youth. If you can equalize all of your negative tension, you will enlarge your life reasonably. These movements are focused on this, self-healing through relaxation, self-medicine through energy. "But any sport would serve for this . . . ," a careful reader would say: well, in theory, any physical activity is positive, but from the point of view from which we have been speaking, sports in general demand too much or burn out certain muscles and therefore the person doing them gets too tired and is not able to rest. For example, if you are one who likes running like crazy every day as if being chased by a huge tiger, I can assure you that all you will accomplish will be to stiffen the muscles in your legs and to damage your spine and your knees due to the rebound from the pavement, not to mention the small pain in your chest that comes from not knowing how to breathe. It is much better, much healthier, and more natural for you to walk. If you do "step" exercises in excess, stepping up and down on a little stool, you will probably damage your knees if you do not die of boredom first. Or we could talk about weight lifting . . . which causes terrible damage to your body. But everyone has to decide what is healthy for them.

The Seamm-Jasani looks to have the weight of the movement to be uniformly distributed across the whole mind/body: legs, thorax, head, neck, sight, fingers, etcetera, with proper breathing techniques and necessary variety, that will produce the real sensation of discharging negativity, along with the awareness of renewal.

Finally, and to keep you readers quiet: if you learn how to breathe and how to coordinate your body and mind, it does not mean that you belong to some religion or special belief. Even today, and despite some murmurings of a "new age," there are still ignorant people who fear that everything new must be feared and persecuted, people whose reactions are always spontaneously neurotic. I would recommend that these people open up their minds. Fear brings tension and if what we are trying to do is enjoy and enlarge our lives, this is far from the best choice; besides, when you learn to enjoy life you no longer pay attention to negativity. If you are negative you are condemning yourself to premature old age, running away from being young. Fear and negativity create a nervous contraction that burns calories unnecessarily, killing more cells in your brain than you can imagine. Persecution of others is a dangerous routine to get into, and do not forget that routine also kills mind.

Always remember that the difference between being young or being old is not in the amount of wrinkles in someone's face—this is merely incidental. The real difference lies in one's mental attitude. I have seen many fifteen, twenty, and thirty year olds who

seemed much older, and many people eighty or older who still remained young.

In summary, and I don't want to bore you too much, I will tell
you that if you would like to shorten your life or your quality of life,
go to extremes: become drug addicts or bohemians, or become
hysterical, bitter, and repressed (personally, I do not know which is
worse). On the other hand, if you want to *live,* to enlarge your life
and its quality, look inside yourself, enjoy every single moment,
and laugh! Because life is too short.

MIND-BODY AND HEALTH: A PROBLEM OF CULTURE

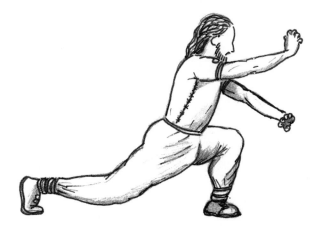

"Every action brings a reaction."

F ROM TIME IMMEMORIAL, human beings have believed
that they have lost the eternal struggle to prolong their lives;
yet, and for this very reason, they have felt a compulsion to devise
ways in which they might lengthen it.

When speaking about eternal youth, it is important to keep in
mind a basic opposition: whether it is better to live longer, full of
tubes, wearing an oxygen mask, with all sorts of doctors hovering
over us waiting to collect on their bills; or to live out the time that
corresponds to each one of us while taking the maximum profit,
the maximum vibration, the maximum of positive energy from it so
that we may reach the dusk of the body with satisfaction, joy, and
a sense of rest as after an amazing meal.

Peasant farmers can be taken as an example, for they often live
a very active life varied in its movements: they rise early in the
morning to milk the cows, water their fields before the sun is at its
height, care for their livestock, cut firewood, walk, walk, and walk

MIND-BODY
AND HEALTH:
A PROBLEM
OF CULTURE

· · ·

some more. This creates, in one way or another, a system of natural and positive exercises.

Every movement has its long-term consequences. If you exaggerate yourself in any one position, the consequences will be negative. For example, spending many hours a day unnaturally bent over sowing or harvesting will cause you pain and, with time, will even deform your spinal column. However, if the work is natural and moderate, with time you will become aware of very positive results.

If you live a balanced life, you will discover the benefits of exercising, of eating good, natural food, of taking walks, and of natural work. With this sort of life you will enlarge your existence in just a couple of years, without medication and a retinue of doctors following you at every step. Often, when men and women from the countryside are ill, they will take local herbs, to which they are already adapted and that they use to compensate any imbalances in their health; after all, chemical medications have their origins in natural herbs. In this case, the people's use of herbs is measured, allowing a natural response from the body and its defenses while encouraging the healthy and necessary interaction between environment, body, and mind. What better than a "peasant death," which takes place at an advanced age yet while the person is still fully active, coming fulminate or in dreams, without time for the suffering of a long and painful agony.

These are rather idealistic examples, for these conditions do not always exist; when these same peasant farmers overwork certain things over others, they face the same consequences that we find in the cities: alcoholism, smoking, stress over constant economic trouble, etcetera. However, from our current point of view, people from the country have a better chance than do those who live in industrialized cities, for nature's wisdom touches those who are willing and able to learn from it. This small course is merely an invitation to return to nature, to simple things, to value work that may seem rougher and more rudimentary, for its benefits are greater than working in an office and living as an executive with cold eyes. This need not blind us, for we must take it only as a part of life and not its entirety. We can untie our tie perfectly, take off our shoes, and go out to sow the earth or we can grab an axe, cut some wood, and build a shed over the weekend.

Human beings are not such specialized machines as they have been depicted by our mistaken modernism: humans are multi-faceted entities with infinite capacities, full of energy, internal light, and a potential strength that can only be expanded. Humans were not born to be brutalized into one specialty. Yet, such specialty can be a path toward achieving great goals so that we might value ourselves and understand that we can excel in every field, with a delicate pencil or a sophisticated computer, with a hammer, shovel, and handsaw, creating positive results with each and every one of them.

Nothing is more boring than a lawyer who speaks only of the law or of her clients, or a doctor who talks about illness all day long: are there no other subjects? Do you want to live longer and better? Change the subject! Stop looking at everything so superficially. Use the materialism; do not let it use you.

At the outset of the industrial era, there was an explosion in the number of people trying to win the race of materialism; to the sorrow of many, the winners turned out to be a very small few. As this era has progressed there has been a slow development (very, very slow) toward an equilibrium in which all can share in the advances of this age. Yet we must never forget the errors that characterized this era, for in one form or another they survive to this day. At the beginning of the industrial era, in England and other similar nations, people were known by appearance, which served as a mark of the city or area from which they came. The specialized machinery and industry of different regions each had its own terrible effect on the workers: those who worked in the coal mines had their hands and faces dyed by it; those who worked in the textile industry could be picked out by their hands; other industries were known by their own specific back problems, lung diseases, etcetera. Human beings became levers, extensions of industry, which brutalized and deformed their bodies and minds. As the medical industry was growing, becoming able to lengthen life, the character of work significantly lowered the quality of it. This is a great contradiction, and from it comes our example of peasant farmers and country people: the need for equilibrium, to not exaggerate what is unnatural for the body.

Nowadays, this exaggerated brutalization that existed in the beginning of the industrial era has supposedly passed; in actuality, it has not. It still affects us in certain ways, and out of this the search for balance and equilibrium is born. For example, a secretary who types a determined amount of hours every day must overwork a few muscles, like the fingers, wrists, and forearms, and also must sit upright in a chair for many hours at a time. This inevitably brings two direct consequences: the numbing of the overworked muscles, and a psychological numbing that occurs as we use only a certain number of static roads in the brain; it is like repeatedly lifting a weight with only one finger. If we take as an example someone who works many hours a day sitting in front of a computer, we will see their sight dimmed, their back injured in the same way as the secretary's. If we look at a senior executive from some company, who has many assistants to carry out different tasks, we could say that he is free of problems; however, the body and the mind form a perfect machine that interacts in constant balance. This person has certain results that he must achieve, goals that might be imposed by his own personal blindness (sorry!) or by his personal ambition, or his company. If he does not accomplish these goals, he becomes more tense, concentrating intensely on this tenseness, while if he does accomplish these goals, he merely aspires to more, this constant ambition tensing him even more. Such "concentration" produces a mental cramp that brings typical consequences: stress, depression, etcetera. Looking at these different examples, we can conclude that those who upset their mental-physical equilibrium will suffer similar consequences.

These days we have extreme cases, such as children committing suicide or falling into drug use, of people trying to find a way out of the pressures that their environment exerts on them. Life itself is a pressure, thus adding more pressure to others and to ourselves is not a good way to lengthen our lives or increase our vitality.

This course, in any case, is not looking to change your lifestyle; it is just advice, just self-discipline through exercises, just a search for equilibrium and for the perfect balancing of our scale, which is inclined toward tensions, frustrations, and routine.

The body and mind of humans create one element, a unity that acts and interacts constantly.

One of the principles of the Seamm-Jasani (or Alayavijnana) is that "every action brings a reaction." Therefore, any physical action, such as moving our hands, walking, or breathing, has its birth in the conscious or subconscious mind. If we move a finger, we should ask ourselves what exactly it is that is moving: is it the muscle, the nerves, the brain, a group of neurons, or what? Without a doubt, its birth is within the brain: doctors have been able to define zones that affect certain parts of the body or the senses, but the initial spark has yet to be deciphered; it will remain so until the concepts behind modern materialistic science have changed. However, based on the Seamm-Jasani, we must look at knowledge gained in practice, which shows that the mind is a field of interaction that casts a large net throughout the rest of the body; thus the mind is not only the mind but also the organs, members, and senses that are both an extension of themselves and are themselves.

After all, any physical movement brings internal consequences: walking establishes a pattern in our brain, but as this is more or less a routine or a preestablished pattern, we say that we do not think when we walk.

Every action brings a reaction, meaning that every physical movement has a psychological counterpart, and vice versa. The basic concept of the Seamm-Jasani is to work with specific types of movements in order to create new fields within our psyche. We are searching for internal awakening, even if it is small; the importance is not in the size of the awakening but in the positive change that begins with harmonious movements. If you feel just a little bit better from these exercises, you have taken the first step toward eternal youth . . . and that is something to be celebrated!

Stage III

THE TWO ARTS

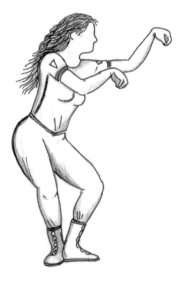

"In the beginning, there was movement."

The Art of Awakening the Body

In the course developed through this book, I must say that, speaking practically, there is a *first art,* which has ten cycles that are related to the idea of reestablishing basic energy. We may call it the Science of *Jass-U,* or the *Art of Revitalizing the Body* (Annamayakosha, in sanskrit). It has three stages of exercises that work as a group and are united into what are called Techniques of Breathing (Pranayama, for East), making thirty-five initial movements. These are developed through physical movements, like a system of exercises or an "anti-gymnastics" that is smooth and harmonious, and accompanied by the corresponding breathing. I call it anti-gymnastics because, even though based in movements that we may find similar to gymnastics, it has an entirely different meaning and execution and does not require its disciple to work himself to death in order to gain positive results.

We also call it the *Art of Awakening,* as our bodies are numbed by our sedentary lifestyle, and because it is a system that is very appropriate for producing the heat, energy, and stretching that are necessary at dawn, after a night during which our muscles have been inactive.

This Art attempts to break the demanding and stressful routine of work and studies. For this, it teaches the student how to activate the different systems that manage the body without becoming bored or unnecessarily tired: we begin with the bone-muscle system, through Fluid Movement (or simple and varied physical exercises); we continue by cleaning the respiratory system through Breathing Techniques. Due to a sedentary lifestyle, we can see our physical response degenerate over the years; with our first steps in this Art, we are trying to reestablish our organism, to awaken and cleanse it internally; to give a general stimulus to the circulatory system, achieving a stability that over time will strengthen the heart and clean out the arteries and the veins, ridding the body of excess fat while lowering cholesterol and uric acid (which is directly linked to psychological states). It could be said that this stage is a real "therapy," because it prevents new illnesses and aids in ridding oneself of many preexisting ones, such as arthritis, diseases of the bones, asthma, ulcers, colon irritation, memory loss, neurosis, depression, migraines, and high blood pressure. It also helps one quit smoking. Even though it may sound amazing, these classes have also shown positive results in people with diseases such as Alzheimer's. It balances the student, who overcomes depressions and decadent states of mind quickly, and as a consequence generally strengthens his or her immune system.

For older people, the physical and psychological works of the movements are very useful. We have seen that women can conquer the negative effects of menopause with physical exercises; the movements developed in this book can be highly beneficial to them, helping them avoid serious problems, such as osteoporosis.

Due to the practical nature of this document, I have summarized the basic movements that embrace simple steps: abdominal, lumbar, and vertebral work in general, along with sight exercises. The pattern of movements in this art is infinitely more extensive, but if our work at this level is good, done with a positive mind once or twice a week, there will be visible and obvious results in our quality of life.

This cycle predisposes and prepares your metabolism so that we may develop, always in the same class, a second art of more complicated movements that we have called, or translated as, *Seamm-Jasani.*

SEAMM-JASANI:
The Art for Eternal Youth

This Art forms the *second art* of the movements, and it is a little bit more complicated than the first because it covers more completely coordination, balance, relaxation, and basic meditation. This is the stage that awakens the life and energy of the Mind and Body, through gentle movements.

This Art is developed through:

1. The Path of Gentle Movement, and
2. The Path of Union: Movement, Breathing, Mind

1. The Path of Gentle Movement

Usually, we execute certain movements, mental as well as physical, that create for us a routine that inevitably causes us problems, as we have explained before. For example, a salesman, a teacher, a student, and a businessman will all eventually become mentally exhausted, due to the routine of pressure, competitiveness, and fear of failure that they deal with every minute of every day. Even though they go to their homes at a certain hour they carry their psychological monotony with them, not allowing their minds to rest and recover satisfactorily from it. This is why such people usually sleep anxious, have a hard time falling asleep, are exhausted and easily irritated when they wake up, and thus why they have stress, ulcers, irritated colons, and all of the "pleasant consequences" of modern life.

The Path of Gentle Movement is based on controlled psychical-physical movement and forces the muscles, nerves, and brain to work in a manner completely outside of the routine that they are used to. When we do what we already know, we are not creating anything in our mental field; in this Art, we do the opposite: as our mind learns new systems of movements we create new paths within it.

Based on this, we will develop sixteen simple coordinative movements that will later be joined with more complete patterns, creating a formula of breathing and meditation that sums to twenty total movements and three steps of meditation. Study the drawings, practice them, and then take one or two classes a week on a schedule that you arrange for yourself.

2. *The Path of Union: Movement, Breathing, Mind*

Another characteristic of this Art is that it looks for constant evolution each and every time you practice it, possessing an enormous variety of movements that create a system of coordination and positive stimulation. This book is a practical summary that can be understood by, and is accessible to, everyone. I have not listed a vast number of movements and coordinations because it is a waste to write about many elements that no one will understand and thus will never practice, leaving this book just another adornment on your beautiful shelf. My intention is solely to give a manageable introduction to an Art that is infinite, both in movements and nature.

The coordinations that are developed here vary and form a dance, or *active meditation,* as body, breathing, mind, and imagination are all working at the same time. What is more important is that everyone can learn it. Through this course you will notice that all the movements have been summarized in three basic *forms,* and at the end of your class you will be able to see how you, without having to be an expert, have been able to execute many movements, joining all of the necessary elements, while discovering great benefits for yourself. Be disciplined, a perfectionist in application, and your achievements will be all the greater; because, after all, you are the only one that can help yourself, as no one can replace your will.

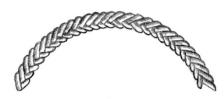

BENEFITS AND ACHIEVEMENTS FOR THE BODY AND MIND

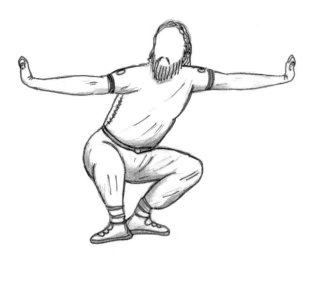

"Nothing that any mind has ever imagined is
impossible to accomplish."

D ID YOU KNOW that human beings use only 10 percent of their cerebral capacity?

In the paths of this teaching, you can speak of psychic effects or a first awakening, because the exercises, breathing techniques, relaxations, and movements put the brain in a state of alertness that includes both of its hemispheres, which are forced to work together. This causes, unconsciously, the awakening of the 90 percent of the brain that is nondeveloped. Work on it and you will see the results. Do you know where the real battle for eternal youth goes on? It happens in your own mind.

Every person, every day, makes certain monotonous movements; as we have already said, they can be physical (for example: getting up every day, driving a car to work in an office, or in the afternoon doing the same, but going back home), or they can be psychological (worrying about bills, about selling more products, passing exams, earning more money, or finding out everything

BENEFITS AND
ACHIEVEMENTS
FOR THE BODY
AND MIND

. . .

about the new car that a coworker just bought). From now on you must only "worry" about important things . . . you!

The simple movements of this science take the student out of his or her routine, in the following ways:

✴   First, it forces him or her to concentrate on movements that are special, but simple.

✴   Second, the student must learn to coordinate and master each technique. This makes them rest physically, even while burning calories. As a consequence, the student can forget his or her worries for a while, an omission or distraction that is highly beneficial, as it allows for the renewal, or recycling, of the psychical and physical energy that moves and motivates the person each day.

✴   Third, the movement causes, on the other hand, a new reaction within the brain that impels it to create new paths, or levels, in both hemispheres, which in the end pushes its development and produces more complete rest. This is when interior awakening begins.

As the student begins to live the classes, he or she will begin to feel small changes, manifesting themselves in:

✴   Tranquility

✴   Energy

✱ Happiness and a great Positivity that can be used in any way the student wants, for personal, professional, or student needs: it is an energy recharger.

Finally, one of the greatest benefits of this Art is that it will help you get to sleep, and it will make you rest when you do it. In general, people do not rest when they sleep, and they wake up tired. It is also hard for many of them to get to sleep at all, so they take drugs, and later on during the day they have to take other chemicals if they want to accomplish anything, and so on. This is lamentable; it is a dark and vicious cycle. These people are just hammering terribly at themselves, without knowing that the true cure has always been inside of them. If you look at this in yourself, you will see that many times you do not sleep well, or when falling asleep you suddenly jump, as if you had tripped; this is because you are charged with negative energy that you have been unable to release due to constant stress during the day. Under these circumstances, the movements of this Art work perfectly: they relax you and help you to *think positively!*

Do your exercises in the mornings and just before going to bed (at least a summary of them) and you will see yourself sleep like a child who has been playing and having fun all day, ready for your "astral voyage" (or conscious dream) in colors and eight dimensions, not an "earthbound trip" in black and white, constantly interrupted and constantly repeating each and every awful situation of the past day. This discussion of astral voyages is a subject for a whole book of its own, and even more, but for now I do not wish to go deeply into this very interesting topic. The important thing is

BENEFITS AND
ACHIEVEMENTS
FOR THE BODY
AND MIND

. . .

that if we are relaxed and have burned the right calories, our night's rest will be 100 percent positive, achieving the objective that "dreaming" be a renovative state, the energizer and main provider of youth for our cells. Sleeping well, achieving the proper biological and internal function of rest, is necessary for the enlargement of vitality, youth, and a positive spirit. Along with food, sleep constitutes, in the old teachings, one of life's sacred elements; it must be cultivated, disciplined, and respected; otherwise, weakness and negative consequences follow quickly.

In recent times, something known thousands of years ago has been rediscovered: that the mind is constantly developing, and that our brains do not necessarily age with our bodies. If we are smart, creative, and restless, our minds will be able to create new paths within themselves and remain young until the end. The brain is one of those mysteries that is not so easy to solve; it is said that certain areas of it influence certain reactions, or parts of the body, and that if damaged it is impossible to re-enliven the corresponding parts or responses. This is not true, for such a small part of the brain is used that it keeps the most unbelievable surprises to itself. The mind is filled with secrets, and this is the reason why doctors have more than once been surprised by positive results from patients technically condemned to paralysis, deficiency, or even death. It is in this moment that science must stop being so narrow-minded and must rid itself of the heavy yoke of its materialistic and dictatorial inheritance from a darker era; it must leave the mentality of the middle ages and join knowledge to wisdom, enlarge its vision of reality and begin to admit that we still have much to learn. I realize that there are many scientists who think that way, and it will depend on them that the advances of a new era are not restricted or misused.

Nowadays, every environment leaves you subject to particularly stressful and competitive situations. We must take time for ourselves. To help us, this Art acts as a psychical-physical relaxant while simultaneously working as a stimulant or mental vitamin, so that we might begin our different activities in a better way, more positively predisposed. Hopefully, in the near future the managers of factories and those in charge of schools will be more conscious, allowing and even encouraging those who work or study under them to have a special time, one that they could dedicate to something so positive and comforting as the Seamm-Jasani.

They would notice results quickly, and the people would rapidly increase in their:

* memory and concentration
* magnetism and creativity
* projection of trust and confidence in themselves.

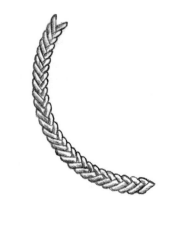

Stage V

THE PRACTICAL
COURSE

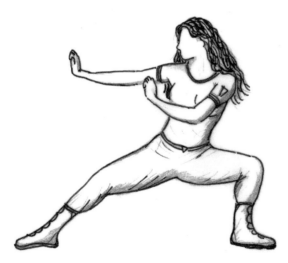

"Science is dreams made into reality."

How to Follow This Course in Practice

Among the many things you will discover through this Art, you will find that the body is a unique, irreplaceable, and precious tool that we must take care of, respect, and conduct in the best possible way. Because of this, you will see that you do not need any sort of implement, weight, rope, spring, electronic masseur, computerized wires plugged who-knows-where, strange meters with television screens, bicycles that go nowhere, or any contraption that looks as if it were a medieval torture device, as if in possessing it you attain some sort of morbid tranquility. You might just want to take my humble advice and save yourself a whole lot of trouble, clean out your basement, and take a look at yourself!

The science developed in this book will teach you that inside of you are all of the natural elements needed for your own advancement, improvement, self-recovery, and equilibrium, and that the body itself (do not forget the mind) is a perfect machine.

Ten thousand years ago, none of these strange "modern" devices existed, and neither did credit cards with which to buy them; yet the human beings from that era who studied this Art lived for 150 years or more, believe it or not.

The drawings in this book are placed in the order that they must be learned and are divided into two separate arts. In the first art, we begin the teaching with simple, basic stretching movements that we use to warm up our own exercise machine: our body. Once this heat has been generated, we can start using the big instrument: our mind.

In order for you to understand more clearly the development of the exercises, they have been numbered in the First Art (Stage VII) from 1 to 35, and in the Second Art (Stage VIII) from 1 to 3 (Meditation Steps) and from 1 to 20 (Meditation in Movement), making a total of fifty-eight movements. The first half includes all of the movements that we call "Movements for Awakening the Body," and the second half is called Seamm-Jasani, or "the Great Wisdom in Practice."

In the beginning, study the primary movements (the Art of Awakening the Body, movements 1 to 35). This whole section is divided into two parts, subdivided into ten cycles, each with different kinds of exercises, forming groups of two to four movements. This is so you can adapt slowly to the movements, for in the beginning it would be impossible for you to do them all: you would get tired trying to understand them and you would not even make an effort to do them. The cycles from the First Art act as a guide, so that you can take examples from each one. Besides, if we consider that you are a normal person from the current era, you haven't had enough time to dedicate to yourself; everything other than you has been a priority. Therefore, do not try to change this all in one day . . . go slowly, step by step, following the chart that has been pedagogically developed in order to familiarize you with Seamm-Jasani, which is the Second Art.

After a few weeks, as you increase the number of movements you can execute, as you understand them and are able to keep them in memory, you will be able to do them in the order that they are described in the text of this book; if you have followed this system, you will be able to do this without problems. Anyway, each movement has different degrees of difficulty that you must understand and regularize, according to how each one feels for you. You do not need to imitate the teacher in our drawings exactly, just do what you can with a medium amount of effort.

As for the amount of time dedicated to each movement, it should be from twelve to twenty seconds or times for each one. You should never exaggerate by trying to eternally extend the time taken on each movement.

After a week, a month, or whenever you think that you are ready, try to have a more complete class by adding movements from the Second Art (movements 36 to 58), and gradually follow the pedagogical chart.

The movements from the Second Art are presented according to their degree of difficulty, and that is why the chart follows their numerical order almost exactly. Not intending to be insistent, I repeat that you should not jump to a new movement without understanding the previous one, because you won't understand the new one, either. The chart provides a program; when having your class review all of the exercises that you already know, then add new ones from each cycle and you will see your class grow longer, as it demands from you greater force, concentration, and mastery.

If you have already mastered all of the movements, follow the order in which they are presented in this book, since this sequence was created specifically to warm up different parts of the body, forming a pattern that facilitates the chain of practice and learning.

If you have not been learning as fast as you had hoped, do not worry, as it is completely normal. Realize that the mind must slowly enlarge its coordinative capacity.

It is probable that it will take from two to five months to really understand everything that is described in this book, to learn the details and execute the movements fluidly. Only when you truly understand what you are doing should you follow the class completely and exactly, because if you try before you are ready you will only be wasting your time, not understanding the real essence of this teaching. You must always follow your own rhythm: there is no room here for competition.

Also, do not get into the bad habit of doing everything quickly and poorly, just to prove that you can do them at all. On the contrary: patience and constancy will be, from now on, your greatest allies.

When uniting the final movements you create patterns that we call *forms,* which summarize all of the previous techniques. If you would like, you can complete this course by executing only the three forms and reviewing them daily, when waking up and before going to bed at night; this will bring many benefits to your state of mind (the main ingredient behind eternal youth). If you would like to continually review the entire class, you can do it once or twice a week, and you will have great success in your rest and energy renewal. But do not review it completely every day.

My advice to all of you is that you begin by studying the movements in this book, looking at the drawings and trying to understand them before you actually do them. It is also very good to practice in nature: on the beach, in the mountains, and, why not, in your place of work, too. In just a few square yards, without bothering anyone, you can execute the movements, relax, recycle your energies, and live a new life! You can do it on your own or you can invite others to join you, but if you want company, make sure that they are people with whom you share similar ideas, otherwise you will get distracted. You can also choose some music to go along with your session, and it does not matter what kind: after all, music takes you to a whole new level of vibration, and as we come closer to equilibrium, we come closer to the music that matches ourselves, spontaneously, without the influence of fashion and talk. Do not think either that it must be some sort of eastern music: vibration is universal; it has neither hemispheres nor sides.

A long session can last forty-five minutes, but if you summarize the movements, you will see that you can review them in less than thirty minutes. Now, if you execute only the forms, you won't need more than five minutes.

Only as a reference and summary have I added a chart that shows how to learn the movements and how to increase them from one session to the next. This chart follows a general method, but each person must adapt it to themselves; this is evident when you consider that your advancement is contingent on your understanding of the previous exercise. Each week the chart covers two sessions (Tuesdays and Thursdays, for example), because there is no need for more; you could also do it only once a week: either way, if you are disciplined, the results will always be positive. Think that, no matter how much you repeat something, it is not necessarily understood, and your mind will always require a break and state of "digestion" for each new piece of information, in order to fully understand it.

In this teaching, patience, constancy, and discipline are fundamental. Work in stages as is indicated, and you will see that, without noticing, you will acquire solid mastery of the movements, and you will see positive, concrete results.

NOTE: Do not even think of doing all of the movements first thing, because you will only choke like a sweet-toothed, spoiled child. The general pattern of development in this book must be quietly digested for at least three months. The best thing is to study the movements as they are meant to be studied.

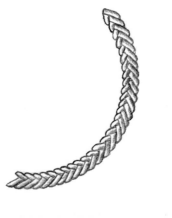

Stage VI

CHART OF PEDAGOGY AND LEARNING

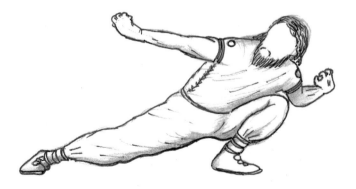

"Discipline is the paintbrush
of the great artist."

T HIS CHART SERVES only as an example. You can edit or extend it as you see fit.

Week 1:
First Art: the following movements will be studied:
"Relaxation" and 1, 4, 5, 9, 12, 14, 19, 23, 27, 33, repeating the Breathing Technique of the Great Circle at the end (movement 4)

The following movements should be gradually added:

Week 2:
First Art: movements 2, 6, 10, 18, 20, 30, 31, and 34
Second Art: movements 36, 37, 38 (Meditations Steps) and 39, 40, 41 (Movements of Active Relaxation)
NOTE: From now on, use the Breathing Technique of the Great Circle to complete each art.

Week 3:

First Art: movements 3, 7, 11, 13, 15, 24, 28, and 32

Second Art: movements 42, 43, and 45

Week 4:

First Art: movements 16, 25, 28, and 29

Second Art: movements 44, 46, 47, 48, and 51

Week 5:

First Art: movements 17, 21, and 22

Second Art: movements 49 (Form 1) and 52

Week 6:

First Art: with movements 8 and 26, we have now completed *Jass-U,* the First Art

Second Art: movement 53

Week 7:

Second Art: movement 50 (Form 2)

Week 8:

Second Art: left-side application of movement 49, and movements 54 and 55

Week 9:

Second Art: movement 56 and the left-side application of movement 50 (Form 2)

Week 10:
Second Art: general review, and the beginning of movement 57 (Form 3: Union)

Week 11:
Second Art: the completion of Form 3

Week 12:
Second Art: Form 3 (completed by the application of the meditation steps), and movement 58: Closing the Circle

The Drawings

In general, the movements are represented by one, two, three, even four or five different drawings. This has been done so the student can better understand the movements. The movements selected are the simplest, most universal, and the easiest to understand through a book, for if we study this teaching in depth, it becomes impossible to explain its details through drawings.

All of the drawings are generally shown from the front and lateral angles, which should clear up any doubts on the correct positions. The arrows indicate direction, and everything else is described in the text. These have been complemented by a few outlines, especially in the breathing and general steps sections.

The author will accept no comment on the drawings, since they were all done by him, personally (along with his noble assistant), and as any amateur draftsman with some respect for himself, he will not suffer any criticism from professionals. Even when specialists offered their assistance, I declined, because I believe that in order to draw the movements of this Art, you must live it and experience it in your own body.

Some Recommendations for Before and After a Class

FOOD: Before a class, it is good not to eat or drink anything for at least two to three hours, depending on one's digestion, though the length of this period will change with the intensity and strength that we apply to our class. The more intensity you put into the exercises, the more strictly you must follow the guidelines on not eating for a certain number of hours.

The body tends to function better on a relatively light stomach, since there is a high concentration of energy in the abdominal area during heavy digestion, which hampers the excellent performance required for such a complete work of the body as ours. It is as if we had a company of one hundred workers, eighty of whom go to lunch exactly when we want to raise our production; obviously the work will be far from optimal and will be delayed or half done.

Another factor in this situation is our individual metabolism and level of personal activity: if we are very active, the food that we consume will be used much faster. Age can also play a role, but as a general rule, it is best to avoid eating for at least a couple of hours before class. So, if you are planning your exercises for the morning, do them before eating breakfast, or, if you prefer the evenings, have class either before dinner or a couple of hours after. After a good class, you will notice that food will taste wondeful and you will enjoy it more than ever, while your body will absorb it much better than before.

This technique, focused over thousands of years on awakening naturalness in each one of us, will help you discover your real "tastes" for foods. These will be the ones that are best for your metabolism, helping you to get rid of habits that over time would have damaged your body. Both eating out of anxiety and not eating at all, out of vanity, are very harmful; perhaps the latter is the worse. What is most important now is that you discover your "middle state."

If, on the other hand, you are hoping by this system of movements to look like an anorexic model in a magazine, you would be much better off returning this book and going straight to the gym, full of strange devices with boob tubes in front and mirrors all over, where you are in very grave danger of dying of boredom! But please take out some medical insurance first that covers both physical and psychiatric treatment, because if you do not end up sick or injured, you will most definitely wind up neurotic and neurasthenic.

The body is a precious, sacred, and very, very delicate instrument, and we must treat it with the utmost respect, harmony, and care. If a competent professional tells you that you are overweight, do not worry; let this Art do its work, which will occur in a slow and natural process, over several months, without negative consequences. Because this teaching helps you to normalize your mind, get rid of anxiety, and direct the burning of calories, you will see that if you remain calm and find an equilibrium within yourself, you will achieve a "middle weight" according to your natural build, age, and shape.

One more thing: please get any ideas of "six-pack" stomachs that you see on TV out of your head. If you were not born with that kind of build, it is best not to worry about that, unless you are a confirmed conceited fanatic who cannot believe in themselves without staring at their image in a mirror or taking steroids. Just stay calm, respect and value yourself the way that you are, relax, and (I must insist!) find your "middle state." That is what you must care about. Personally, I still have my favorite "love handles" and I am not planning on getting rid of them any time soon.

PLACE AND OUTFIT: Our art speaks of internal heat, therefore it is a good idea to look for warm places in which to do the movements. It can be any kind of room—bedroom, office, etcetera. We can also look for a quiet place in the park or at the beach, but we must always be warm. Obviously, if you live in a warm area of the planet or if it is summer where you are, you will not need too many layers.

As for what to wear, it can be anything that makes you feel comfortable. And please, you do not need to look like a ninja and you do not need to wear some special color. If you are going to review all of the movements, you are going to sweat quite a bit, and it is much better for you to wear comfortable sports clothes, preferably those made out of cotton. If you are only going to review the breathing techniques and basic forms, you will see that you don't need special clothes.

However, it is advisable (though not an obligation) that, in order to have a good class, you forget about your watch, jewels, rings, chains, wires, earrings, nails through your nose, etcetera, because you will see that, aside from dropping a couple of pounds, you will become more fluent in your movements without being distracted, strangled, or scratched by your jewelry. (Besides, in the old teachings, metal is just a symbol of "delay" in a person's energy field, which manifests itself most clearly in matters concerning the expansion of energy, which is the primary concern of the Art taught here.) Now, if you have one or more tattoos on your body do not worry, they will not be erased by this Art; on the contrary, the only risk that you are taking is that you might start to value yourself for who you really are and not for what it is that you carry (or for what you have painted on).

As for privacy, it is always best to find a situation where you can be as concentrated as possible in the execution of the movements. Having a good partner is no problem at all . . . it is up to you!

AFTER CLASSES: If your session is going to be long and you are planning to review all of the movements, it is always good advice to take a hot shower afterward. Do not take a cold shower because, despite what you may have heard, that sort of temperature change is completely destructive to our aims. If it is hot outside, you will obviously use cooler water, but never inflict sudden and drastic temperature changes on your body: it is like a glass made of crystal. If you change its temperature suddenly from hot to cold it will break, and I do not want to see this happen to any of you.

I know that there are many who hold the opposite belief, but please be cautious and listen to my advice: the human body belongs to heat, and if you want to completely relax yourself after a class, take a bath and add a handful of sea salt. This will be very good for you and will renew you, as will bath salts, if you have them. If you like, as I do, natural herbs, you can add a bit of boiled laurel to your bath. You will find this very relaxing.

RECOMMENDATIONS IN CASE OF INJURIES: In general, this Art is adaptable to every person and does not contain contraindications. If you have serious problems in your spine or back, you should be cautious with some of the movements, especially those concentrated on the abdominal zone. Always do what you can without pushing yourself too hard; do not exaggerate the movements and make sure to pay attention to the chart at the beginning of this chapter, meaning that you should not try to do everything in the first day. Follow a slowly expanding regimen while you learn and your body will adapt slowly. This is very important.

Whatever the case, the author does not take responsibility for irresponsible people. If you really feel concerned about these movements because of your heart, spine, pregnancy, or any other reason, make sure to consult your physician first and follow his or her recommendations.

AGE: Age does not in any way limit your capacity to follow this ancient Art. Actually, age has its advantages, from two extreme points of view. First of all, someone very young has the advantage of physical and psychical flexibility, which will allow him or her to adapt quickly to the cycle of movements; however youth also has the disadvantage of limited concentration and dedication, which are the greatest barriers facing a child or adolescent attempting to study these movements. On the other hand, an adult, while most likely not as flexible as a child, has the advantage of having won the patience necessary for dedication and concentration in life, which for this teaching is a very important skill. Thus, age really does not matter at all: what matters is internal energy!

If there are any movements that you cannot do or do not understand, just go on to the next one. With time you will be able to understand and do all of them. If, on the other hand, you cannot exactly imitate the positions as they appear in the drawings, then adapt them to your body, build, or limitations by shortening the time you spend in difficult positions. With time you will be able to execute them better, which is important. But never demand more of yourself than you actually can give.

As for the suggestion that this Art might be better suited to either men or women, one should not be foolish. That is only a prejudice and just as any other macho or feminist prejudice, it is just plain silly. For poor, traumatized humanity now is the time to learn balance, mutual respect, and to accept the fact that we all have within ourselves the conditioning necessary to evolve, and we each have our own way to do it.

A Secret Art: For thousands of years the Art for Eternal Youth has been kept secret, and I am taking a risk in teaching the basic patterns of its development and application. In any case, the secret will be kept, since those who do not want to learn and who do not have the discipline to learn will never learn, though you can show them all you want.

Ignorance blinds the vision of curious onlookers. For such people, all knowledge is hermetic, secret, or impossible to understand, just as it was impossible to fly or to study the human body during the Middle Ages; thus it has always been and thus it shall remain.

From a different point of view, what I present here is only the tip of the iceberg, and this course is simply the summary of two different sciences whose development is so extensive that they would require 1,008 books in order to be understandable. The *Seamm-Jasani* is the translation of an ancient system whose original name belongs to a language unknown to both East and West. This Art is one of twenty-eight disciplines that embrace the complete development of energy, vitality, harmony, self-control, magnetism, bony or osseous defense, internal strength, and mind, for all of which time, dedication, and great constancy are necessary, not simply the reading of a manual.

Make good use of the knowledge that is contained here. As a compiler of this book, I consider myself a humble professor and seeker: we all share the same road.

If you search and persevere, you will see that the appropriate answer will always come.

I give you a Great Positive Energy
and I welcome you!
Learn, enjoy this teaching,
and have the greatest successes!

Stage VII

THE FIRST THIRTY-FIVE FUNDAMENTAL MOVEMENTS

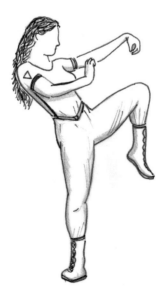

"Self-awareness begins with the body."

First Art:

Jass-U
The Art of Awakening the Body

All of the movements that we are about to describe form the First Art, a set of simple yet dynamic exercises that you will use to awaken your body. Most generally, it is divided into two parts: Standing and Seated, respectively. The first part includes movements 1 through 18, grouped in cycles one through six, according to type. The second, seated part includes movements 19 through 35, grouped in cycles seven through ten.

Most of the drawings show both the frontal and lateral view, in that order, to show most movements from both perspectives. Obviously, the drawings are in the same order as the movements.

Now, study them, understand them, review them, work with them, and let's *wake up!*

First Part:
Standing Movements

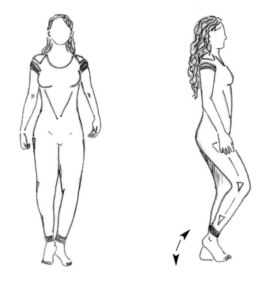

General Basic Movement: Relaxing and Loosening Up

Gently relax your arms and legs (we will usually do this between movements to release tension and keep ourselves from getting tired; when we say "relax," this is what we mean). Walk in place, gently and comfortably moving your arms and legs in order to release the basic tensions from your extremities. Clear your mind and imagine yourself walking through beautiful fields.

First Cycle

1. Forward Arm Stretch

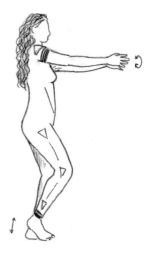

This is the first movement of the first cycle, and it is based on a very simple mechanism. Continue to relax your legs (pretending to walk just as before), while extending your arms in front of you with your fingers pointing out, turning them as if turning a lightbulb in and out of a socket on the wall in front of you (circular movement to the front, inside, and outside).

All of these movements will channel the energy from your extremities, each in a different way. Now the muscles are working in a circular pattern, twisting. Your legs should always remain moving.

The drawing shows a lateral view of the movement, as does the detail of the hand.

Count to 12 and then begin the next movement.

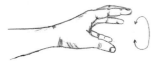

2. Lateral Arm Stretch, with Lowering

Continue to relax as described above, while extending your arms to both sides and making the same movements with your hands that you did in the previous exercise, that of twisting a lightbulb, except that now the sockets are at your sides.

To begin to give life to your lower zone, vertically lower yourself a little bit, bending at the knees as if you were going to sit down, then bringing yourself back up. If you want to complicate this movement a little, try to lower yourself some more before going back up very slowly. At the beginning it is enough if you only lower yourself a little, bending your knees just a bit. Even though this may seem easy, your legs will begin to work in a different way than they are used to.

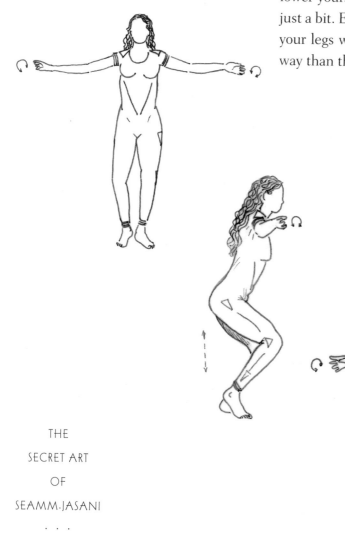

3. High Arm Stretch, with Lowering

Continue relaxing. Now raise your arms straight above your head while continuing the same movement with your hands, as if twisting a lightbulb, this time with your hands pointing at the ceiling. Now lower yourself, just as in the previous exercise.

The top two drawings describe the movement of the hands, while the bottom two add the movement of lowering yourself with your legs.

If properly executed, this movement will make you feel as if you are making a great effort with your arms; do not worry, this is completely normal.

Count to 12 and continue.

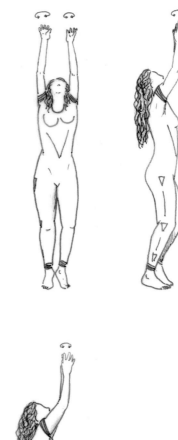

4. Breathing Technique of the Great Circle

This movement requires extra-special attention and observation as you learn it, as the understanding of this breathing technique is related to, and vital for, all the rest of the movements.

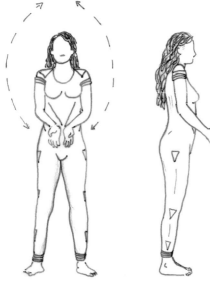

**Figure 1a
(frontal)**

**Figure 1a
(lateral)**

The breathing technique (or Pranayama, for East) will be explained in three stages: the first will show the physical movements involved, called the External Movement; the second analyzes the position of the breathing tracts as well as the sound required for proper execution of the technique, all of which is called the Internal Movement. Finally, we will gather both internal and external stages. After this we will discuss the objectives for and benefits of a correct breathing technique.

FIRST: Stand normally, your back and shoulders straight but without exaggeration, with your feet about seven inches apart. Put your hands in front of your body as shown in figure 1a, just a bit out in front, and then move them in a smooth and harmonious circle as shown in figure 1b, until your hands are flat and above your head, as in figure 1c.

As you move your hands up, lean your body slightly back in order to produce the maximum natural extension of the chest wall. Then return your hands, with the same motion, to where they began, and you have traced the same circle in reverse.

Make sure to pay special attention to the drawings, as they show three stages of the circle: beginning, middle, and its fullest extension, from both the frontal and lateral views. The return is identical.

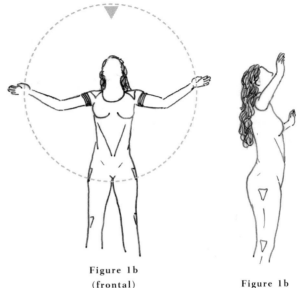

Figure 1b
(frontal)

Figure 1b
(lateral)

SECOND: In this part we see in detail the position and flow of our respiratory and breathing system.

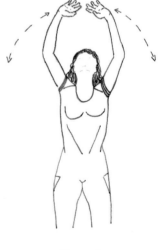

Figure 1c

THE INHALATION: Begin by putting your tongue in your palate and inhaling through the nose. You will feel a little pressure in your nasal cavities as a natural result (this is shown in figure 2a with small arrows). When inhaling, we produce a specific sound (nnnsss . . .) by applying a slight force to the entering air. The sound must be loud, audible from at least five or six feet in a quiet place. This is important, for it is by the audible sound that we know

· · ·

85

when the execution of the breathing technique is correct. This is as the old teachings say: "Know the sound of your body, know the sound of life."

You must also try to produce this sound for as long as possible, forcing the air to enter as slowly as possible, in order to filter and heat it enough for its later "digestion," while you attempt to expand your chest as much as you can while also expanding your stomach, which will work to lower the diaphragm, as in figure 2a. Now comes what we call the Containment.

THE CONTAINMENT: You must hold the air, with all of its nutrients, for about five seconds, while keeping your hands still above your head.

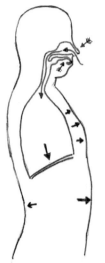

Figure 2a

THE EXHALATION: This is the third phase of breathing. For it, you must use a high exhalation, as follows: remove your tongue from your palate and exhale through the mouth, rounding the lips and forcing the air along the throat, gently scratching it and making a "hhhaaa . . ." sound. The natural pressure of this phase is exerted in the throat, as shown by the small arrows in figure 2b. With this, we are cleaning out the dirt, the small particles of dust that settle in our breathing tracts. As the lips are rounded, the sound of this exhalation is a combination of "a" and "o," and this sound also must be audible at least five or six feet away. If it is inaudible, it will not result in the benefits that we seek.

Concentrate on the details, breathe well, and with practice you will see positive results.

When inhaling and exhaling, you must extend the movement as much as possible each and every time. Even though it is normal that in the first sessions your lung capacity will be small, you will discover with time that the lungs are muscles and can be developed, stretched, and enlarged just as any other, except that in the case of the lungs the benefits are noticeable throughout your entire body.

This exercise will have the same effect on you as it would if you replaced a dirty carburetor in a car with a brand-new one: now that it is clean, its capacity is greatly increased and, with such modifications over time, your VW Bug will be turned into a race car.

THIRD: Now that you understand the internal and external aspects of our breathing, we will gather them together and practice the entire technique, so that we may use it with all of the movements. Follow this order:

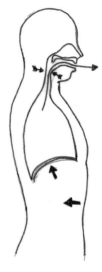

Figure 2b

1.   Standing normally, with your hands as they are in figure 1a, put your tongue in your palate and inhale, making the nasal "nnnsss . . ." sound while slowly raising your arms, tracing a circle with your hands (figure 1b) until, as they are directly above your head (figure 1c), you stop inhaling.

2.   Once your hands are above your head and you have stopped inhaling, contain the air in your lungs for about five seconds, while keeping your hands up. Your thorax and diaphragm are now completely extended (figure 1c).

3.   Take your tongue out of your palate, round your lips, and exhale over the back of your throat, scratching it while lower-

ing your arms over the same circle that you raised them. Breathe out slowly, making the "hhhaaa . . ." sound with your throat, your arms moving as slowly as your breath, returning to their initial position just as the sound stops. Then, rest.

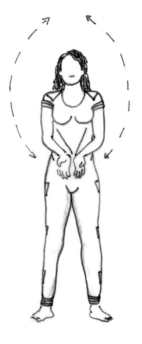

This technique must be repeated two or three times. It is also a form of rest, and a good way to release tension and relax in bad situations. If your situation is negative, breathe this way and you will feel relieved; if you are at work about to have a "simple" discussion with your boss about "this and that," execute this breathing technique and you will find yourself feeling more confident, calm, and relaxed. Take the same advice if you have a business appointment, if you are a student facing an exam, etcetera. Always keep this breathing technique in mind, as it will help you clear your mind, calm down, and escape a nervous mental state.

Someone who has increased his or her lung capacity and has become skillful in this exercise will trace the circle very slowly, both when inhaling and exhaling. A beginner, however, will try to do it quickly. This is a measurement or a test of your lung capacity: the circle will tell the truth. But remember that this is not about competition, that you must just relax and do your best, and that over time you will slowly achieve more and more.

With this, we have learned the three basic stages of life: birth, plenitude, and dilution (inhalation, containment, and exhalation), from which no one escapes. Even though we may feel big or important, even though we may have heaps of money or believe ourselves rich, even if we see ourselves as gods on Earth or adore our physical selves with supreme vanity, we are inevitably subject to that principle and its three stages. If you think about this breathing technique, it becomes a symbol of existence that teaches us harmony with ourselves, that teaches us to flow and to be humble. Youth and old age are just physical cycles; birth, plenitude, and dilution are quick stages in comparison with the mind, which has a superior state of vibration with its own birth, expansion, and dilution, which are eternal when compared with our bodies.

If you enjoy living, begin to look at yourself and stop practicing limitless ambition, intolerance, and persecution; you will see that the mind lives forever and that it will unconsciously give order to your body so that it might remain with her for as long as possible.

Objectives and Other Benefits of a Correct Breathing Technique

The importance of breathing is obvious to us all. This technique attempts to enrich something that we are used to doing without thinking. What our Art teaches is that the body is in constant combustion, that the mind is a great bonfire. Giving more oxygen to the mind increases that combustion, and the breathing technique helps us with this. First, it increases lung capacity, which allows more oxygen into the lungs and thus into the blood, the rest of the body, and especially into the brain. With more oxygen, the internal flame grows and the mind relaxes, becomes comfortable, positive, and open to any work or effort, be it mental or corporeal.

At the same time, this breathing technique helps to cleanse all of the passageways in your body, cleaning the nasal passages and the throat as it also helps you, in a natural and indirect way, to quit smoking. You will feel, in just a few weeks of regular practice, that you do not need to smoke as much as you used to. Your cravings will reduce more and more until this habit disappears, without anxiety or problems.

From now on, each exercise will be accompanied by the same inhalation and exhalation, following the same basic pattern with the tongue and with the scratching of the throat. It is normal if this technique produces a little dizziness in the beginning—this is because you are feeding your body a new "food," one that it is not used to. It is the same as eating a lot after having starved for a while.

When you feel that you have mastered this technique, you can continue with the rest of the movements. In each of them you must use the same technique of inhalation and exhalation, sometimes with small variations that will be explained when they arise.

In general, this breathing technique should be executed twice, before continuing with the rest of the movements.

5. *Pushing Forward*

Begin by continuing to relax your arms and legs. Stop and draw your arms to your sides (figure 3a), then push them forward (figure 3b) as if pushing a large imaginary object.

Always keep your back straight and remember to inhale while pushing forward (putting your tongue in your palate). Exhale when returning your arms to your sides, remembering here to round your lips. Relax your arms and legs between each "push," then repeat the movement.

When executing this movement, use your imagination and picture yourself expelling something from your body, liberating yourself from it.

Count to 12 and continue with the next movement.

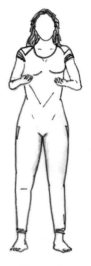

**Figure 3a
(frontal)**

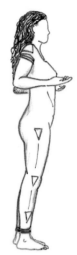

**Figure 3a
(lateral)**

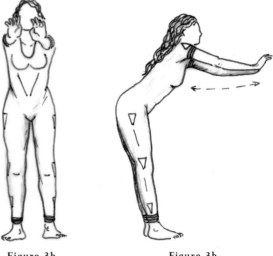

**Figure 3b
(frontal)**

**Figure 3b
(lateral)**

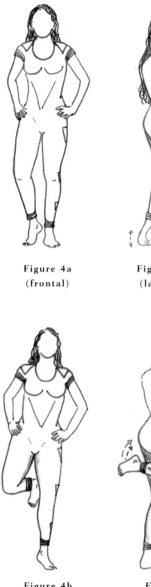
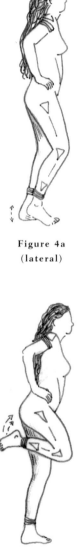

Figure 4a
(frontal)

Figure 4a
(lateral)

Figure 4b
(frontal)

Figure 4b
(lateral)

6. *Heel Up*

Relax your legs with your hands on your hips (figure 4a). Now kick your heel backward, bending your knee and touching your buttocks with your heel (figure 4b). You should kick up twice, quickly, inhaling with each kick (nnnsss . . . nnnsss . . .), and exhale (hhhaaa . . .) while more slowly lowering your leg. You can begin by doing this one leg at a time through the whole cycle, but as you become more proficient you can try alternating legs, one and then the other.

This is a simple movement that many people use as a standard exercise, except that here we are complicating it with the two short inhalations as you bring your heel up, as shown in the drawings.

Count to 12 (with each leg) and go on to the next movement.

7. *Swimming to the Front*

Relax in the normal manner, then bring your hands to your sides, as shown in the first drawing. Lean a little to the front and move your hands forward, right over left, with your palms up. Lean forward (keeping your back straight) as you continue to extend your arms. When your arms are at their fullest extension, turn your palms to face outward and move your hands horizontally, as if swimming, tracing two circles, moving your body back to a normal standing position as your hands come back to their starting position.

Relax again, then bring your hands to your sides and repeat the whole sequence.

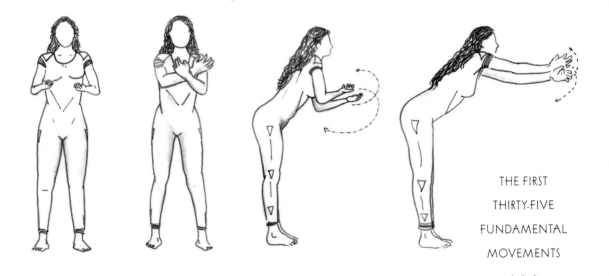

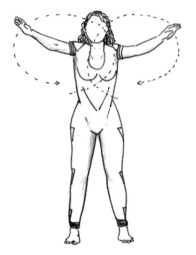

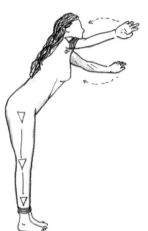

Pretend you are swimming in an imaginary ocean: the waves refresh us, gently touching us while we swim. This makes us feel happy, relieved, and new—use your imagination!

Execute this movement twelve times and continue.

8. *Crouching and Pushing*

Begin by relaxing your arms and legs. Then bring your hands to your sides, as in the previous exercises and as in the drawing, with your feet shoulder-width apart. Then crouch quickly, separating the knees and with the feet nearly touching, as if you were falling straight down. The very last part of the crouch should be repeated twice, as if you were bouncing just a little, and you should breathe in twice (nnnsss . . . nnnsss . . .), once the first time your drop and another on the bounce. Exhale once (hhhaaa . . .) while rising back to the original position, then relax again.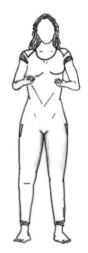

While you are "falling," push your arms twice to the front, co-ordinated with your breathing and crouching. Bring them back to your sides as you rise again, then relax. Then, repeat the whole movement again from the beginning.

Even though it may seem simple, this movement has a certain difficulty to it. It is better if you do not try to execute this move-ment exactly as it appears in the drawings at first, but try it out gently until you feel that you un-derstand it and it feels comfort-able (how to bend your knees, push, and straighten your body). With time and practice, you will perfect it.

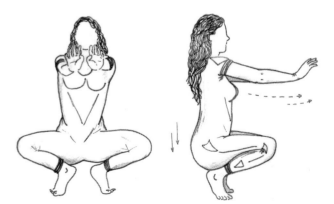

Repeat this twelve times, and go on to the next exercise.

. . .

9. *Two Circles*

Continue to relax your legs and put both hands in front of you, with your arms bent (figure 5a). Now, keeping your palms flat and facing forward, form two circles (figures 5b–e), not too big and not too small, as if washing a window. Remember to continue moving your legs the whole time.

In our minds and on our faces we cultivate a simple happiness, an expression of sympathy and joy while making these circles. With a little effort you can forget the whole world . . . expand your positive thoughts while doing this strange dance of life and you will see it relieve you of any stressful thoughts.

Make twelve to fifteen circles and continue.

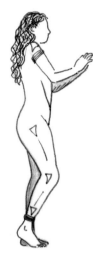

Figure 5a (lateral)

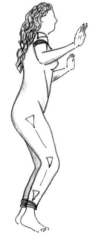

Figure 5d (lateral)

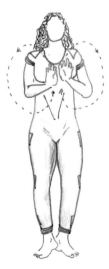

Figure 5b (frontal)

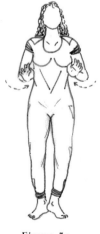

Figure 5e

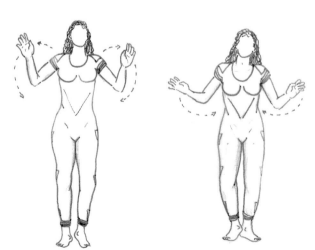

Figure 5c   **Figure 5d**

10. Relaxing the Forearms and Wrists

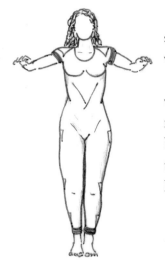

Begin by standing still, your arms at your sides with your forearms in front, as if you were sitting in an armchair (figure 6a).

Now bring your forearms back, with your wrists limp, as if they were tired and could not resist (figure 6b). Move your arms back twice, breathing in (nnnsss . . . nnnsss . . .) each time, and then bring them back with a long exhale (hhhaaa . . .).

Count to 12 and go on.

Figure 6a

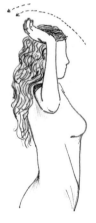

Figure 6d

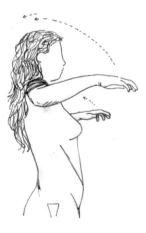

Figure 6b

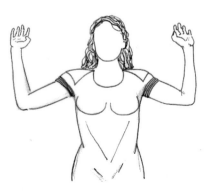

Figure 6c

11. Relaxing the Wrists

Stand normally, with your arms in front of you, making fists and bending your wrists. Keep your arms still as you swing your fists front to back, quickly, inhaling and exhaling at your own pace.

Be conscious of the weight of your fists as you swing them, and as you understand this movement better swing them faster.

Count to 12 as you breathe, then continue.

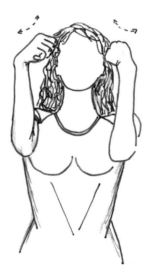

12. *Bending the Knees: Frontal*

Initial position: with your feet together (figure 7a), put both hands on your knees, keeping your back straight. Bend your knees forward in two short movements (figure 7b), almost standing on your toes, and inhale with each one (nnnsss . . . nnnsss . . .). Exhale when returning to the initial position.

Count to 12, then relax your arms and legs.

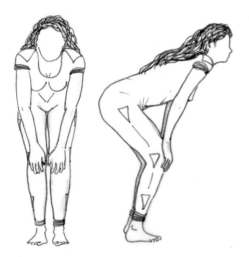

Figure 7a
(frontal and lateral)

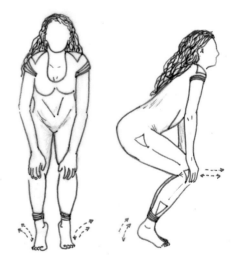

Figure 7b
(frontal and lateral)

13. Bending the Knees: Lateral

Begin in the same position as the last movement (12, figure 7a). Instead of bending your knees forward, move them to the side in two short movements (figure 7c), inhaling twice (nnnsss . . . nnnsss . . .). Work on leaning your feet and ankles out as slightly as possible.

Start off with one side, inhaling twice, exhaling once in the middle, then inhaling twice on the other side, and so on.

Do twelve movements on each side and then relax your arms and legs again.

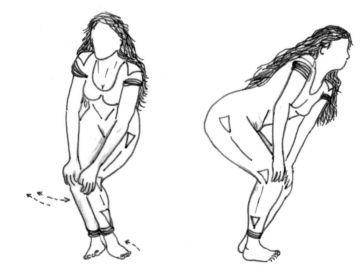

Figure 7c
(frontal and lateral)

14. *Bending at the Waist, Two Times*

Initial position: stand normally, with your hands at your sides, as in figure 8a. Bend over, lowering your torso with your arms straight and down (figure 8b), and the palms of your hands facing up. Do not bend your knees.

Try to touch the floor (though you should not force anything) with two short extensions while you inhale twice (nnnsss . . . nnnsss . . .). Then come back to the initial position. Bring your hands to your sides with two short movements, accompanied by two exhalations (hhhaaa . . . hhhaaa . . .).

Immediately repeat the downward movement, repeating the two downward hand movements and the double inhale, then again straighten your body while exhaling twice, without losing continuity.

Use your imagination with this movement, and we will pretend to be a machine, or the engine of a

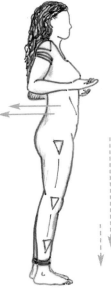

Figure 8a

train: slowly it speeds up while our body stays firm and in control. As you feel more confident with this exercise you can move faster, going up and down, inhaling twice and exhaling twice with two short extensions of our arms. Now you are strong, your engine has broken through its inertia and every time we move faster and faster.

THE FIRST

THIRTY-FIVE

FUNDAMENTAL

MOVEMENTS

. . .

After twelve to twenty seconds we slow down calmly, relax, and finally stop.

With this movement we have broken up our solid energy and forced it to rush through our whole body. Always remember not to overexert yourself, and make sure that you keep it interesting for you; everyone needs to work according to his or her own body.

Now relax your arms and legs normally and continue with the following movements.

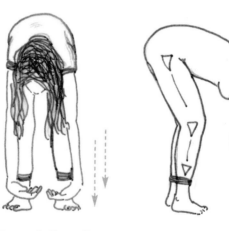

Figure 8b (frontal)   Figure 8b (lateral)

15. Stretching Downward

Begin this movement in the same position as the last, standing up straight with your arms at your sides. Now slowly lower your torso while inhaling, and when you are down with your arms hanging, exhale once. Inhale again, stretching more and more as you try to touch the ground with the backs of your hands. You should feel a gentle heat or tickling in the backs of your arms and head.

Exhale once as you return slowly to the initial position. You have just forced a lot of blood into your head and upper extremities, so a little dizziness is completely normal.

This technique is special and if you like you can do it every morning to help you awaken and renew your brain. You will blush quickly, having just received an excellent stimulant and vitamin.

Do this three times, then go on to the next movement.

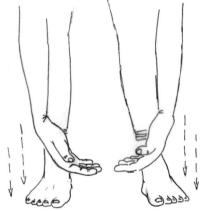

16. Stretching Upward

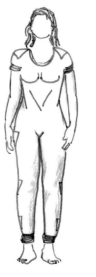

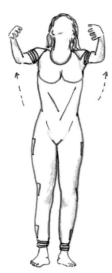

Stand normally with your arms relaxed at your sides. Raise your arms slowly above your head as you inhale. When your arms are fully straightened, exhale, but keep them above your head. Then inhale again, trying to touch the ceiling, straightening your body as much as you can, trying to touch the sky and beyond. Now lower your arms slowly, exhaling.

It is normal again to feel a little heat or tickling in your upper extremities: don't worry, because it is just your body waking up.

Stretch three times and continue.

Figure 9a

Figure 9b

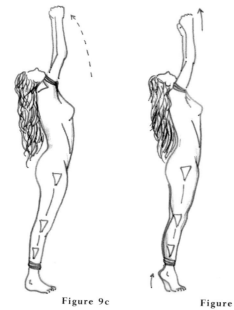

Figure 9c

Figure 9d

17. Stretching Your Back

Stand normally, but put your arms behind your back, each hand grasping the opposite forearm, as the drawing shows. Make two short movements to the front, inhaling (nnnsss . . . nnnsss . . .) and bending your back just a little. Then return to your initial position, exhaling once (hhhaaa . . .).

This is a delicate exercise that you must do gently, without forcing the movement too much. You are working with your spine, and you have to treat it with all possible respect and care, as it is what ties us to the Earth, and to truth.

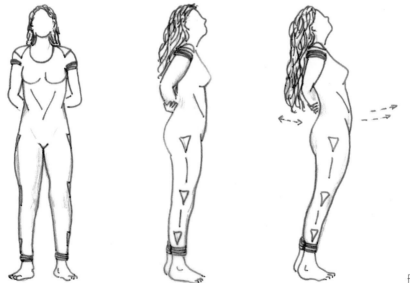

THE FIRST

THIRTY-FIVE

FUNDAMENTAL

MOVEMENTS

. . .

105

Personally, I feel awful when I see young athletes who are full of vitality doing incredible things with their spines, because they have no idea the harm they are causing themselves. With time, especially if they continue to abuse their spines over a long period (not to mention some of those yoga exercises that try to turn a person into a circus freak!), they will suffer terrible consequences.

Youth is ephemeral and old age is far too long . . . therefore, it is much better to live a balanced youth in order to have a balanced and complete maturity where you don't have to pay the bills for the abuses of your youth. When people force their backs unnecessarily with any type of exercise, the harm done is terrible, especially for older people who get overzealous about these activities. If you care about your back and take care of it, this movement is not only harmless, it is beneficial. If you are careful, you will find only positive results.

Do this about twelve times (carefully!) and continue.

18. Tracing a Circle

Stand with your legs far apart and your hands pulled in to your sides, palms facing up. Begin by bringing your arms to one side, as if pushing an imaginary object. Then trace a wide and smooth semicircle in front of your body, keeping your arms in one horizontal plane. When you reach the other side, bring your hands

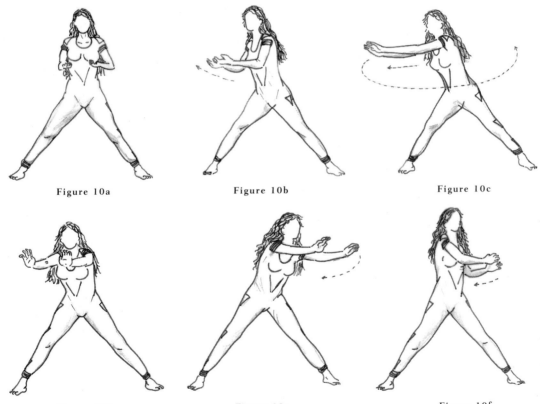

Figure 10a

Figure 10b

Figure 10c

Figure 10d

Figure 10e

Figure 10f

· · ·

back to your sides. Make sure you inhale (nnnsss . . .) from the beginning all through the circle and exhale as you are bringing your hands back to your sides (hhhaaa . . .).

Repeat the exercise, but in the opposite direction. Alternate directions one for one, making sure to inhale and exhale each time. Pay attention to the drawings: they show the movement from beginning to end and should clear up any confusion you might have (figures 10a–f).

Use your imagination and pretend, for example, that you want to embrace a whole lot more, so expand yourself and enjoy this simple and healthy movement. Repeat it slowly, about twelve times.

With this movement we have completed the standing exercises, and now we move to the floor.

(In order to complete the whole cycle of standing movements, execute the Breathing Technique of the Great Circle twice.)

Second Part:
Movements on the Floor

This section of movements does not need to be done on the floor: you can also do them sitting in your bed or wherever you feel comfortable. Keep in mind that you have to adapt the movements to your body, not your body to the movements. You do not need to follow them to the letter. Some of them have alternate positions that you should use if the given positions feel uncomfortable.

THE FIRST
THIRTY-FIVE
FUNDAMENTAL
MOVEMENTS

. . .

109

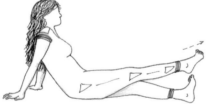

19. Knee to Shoulder, Two Times

Sit down with your legs straight, your arms on the floor behind you, straight and supporting your weight, as shown in the drawings. Now bend your leg and bring your knee to your shoulder in two short movements, inhaling twice (nnnsss . . . nnnsss . . .), then straighten your leg in front of you as you exhale once (hhhaaa . . .). Now rest. When extending your leg, try to keep your feet in the position shown in the drawing: foot pointed forward and toes bent back, like a ballerina. Now repeat, but with the other leg.

Do this twelve times with each leg and continue with the next movement.

NOTE: To relax the legs between movements, sit in the same position with your legs extended and move them slightly, one and then the other as shown in the drawing. This sort of relaxing movement should be used any time you need to, especially after having been in the same position for a long time.

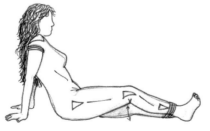

20. Stretching Two Times to the Front

Begin in the same way as the previous movement, but now bring both arms forward, trying to reach the space above your feet, inhaling twice with two short movements of the arms (nnnsss . . . nnnsss . . .), and exhaling once (hhhaaa . . .) as you put your hands back on the floor.

Execute this movement twelve times, then relax your legs as indicated in the last movement.

Now go on to the following movement.

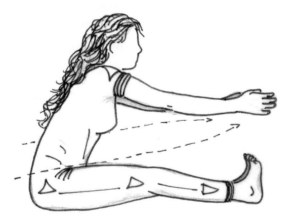

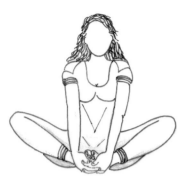

21. High Butterfly Position

Seated with your feet together, hold your feet with your hands interlaced. Remember to always keep your back straight, and if you can't quite do that just put your feet together and sit with your hands flat on the floor behind you (see alternate position). Now, try to bring your knees as close to your body as you can while inhaling once (nnnsss . . .). Hold them there for a moment before you let them back down, slowly exhaling as you do. As you are exhaling, you should feel deep relief, as if you were pushing all of your worries out of your body. If you concentrate on this, you will see its benefits.

Do this movement twelve times, then continue with the next one.

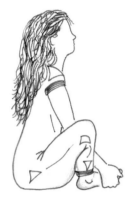

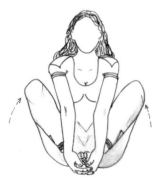

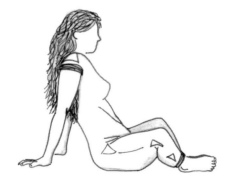

alternate position

22. Low Butterfly Position

The initial position is the same as in the last movement, whether you like the standard or alternate form better. Now, try to open up your knees, lowering them as much as you can while you inhale (nnnsss . . .). Then rest, exhaling as you bring your knees back (hhhaaa . . .). When you exhale, think about the relief and serenity of quietness . . . these relaxing thoughts will calm your whole body.

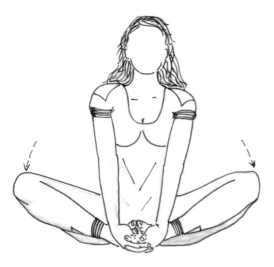

THE FIRST
THIRTY-FIVE
FUNDAMENTAL
MOVEMENTS

. . .

113

23. On Your Back, Lifting Your Head Twice

Lie extended on your dorsal ulna (with your back completely extended on the floor and your shoulders lifted slightly). Make fists with your hands and hold them over your stomach. Now lift

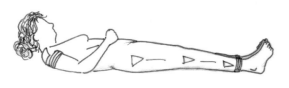

your head up from the floor, trying to make your chin touch your chest in two quick movements, inhaling each time (nnnsss . . . nnnsss . . .). Exhale each time as you bring your head back twice (hhhaaa . . . hhhaaa . . .), making sure not to hit your head on the floor!

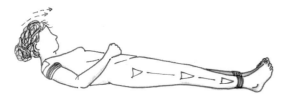

Continue bringing your head up and down, always in two short movements, inhaling and exhaling.

This is a great exercise for your neck muscles, but be careful and make sure that you keep your back on the floor, as this movement is working your head, neck, and stomach.

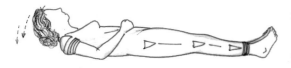

Do this twelve times, then rest for a minute, lying flat on the floor. You can use your fingers to gently relax the back of your neck.

24. On Your Back, Lifting One Leg

Lying on your back as before, lift your head to look over your body and hold your hands in fists over your stomach. Now lift your right leg straight up, inhaling twice (nnnsss . . . nnnsss . . .) while making two short movements when your leg is at the top of its arc. Now lower your leg, exhaling twice (hhhaaa . . . hhhaaa . . .) with two short movements just above the floor. Do not let your leg touch the floor. Remember to always keep your toes flexed back at you.

Repeat this exercise twelve times with one leg, then twelve times with the other.

If you do this exercise properly, you will be working with three major zones of your body: your neck, your stomach, and your legs, all without putting pressure on your back.

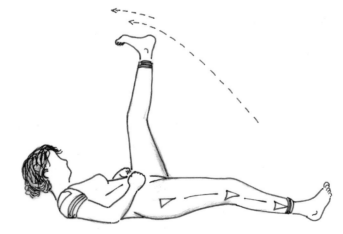

25. Fingertips Out Front, with Abdominal Work

Sit up with your legs straight out in front of you. Keep them together. Now, hold your arms out in front of you and work with your fingertips, continually opening and closing them (as in the drawings). Keeping your back straight, start to lean back a little, then a little more, and then some more. This will work your stomach muscles.

If you want to feel more tension in your stomach, you can lean back a little bit farther, but don't abuse yourself with this movement. Try for a medium level of exertion.

Count slowly to 8 (or 12), then rest.

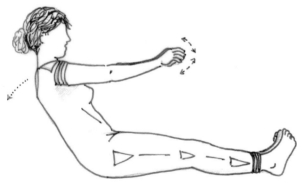

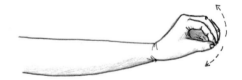

26. On Your Stomach,
Lifting the Top Third of Your Body

Lie down on your facial ulna (with your abdomen on the floor), with your chest raised, supporting yourself on your elbows and holding your head and thorax so that you feel comfortable. From this position inhale twice (nnnsss . . . nnnsss . . .) while lifting both your head and wrists up in two short movements. Return to your initial position as you exhale once (hh-haaa . . .).

Repeat this movement about twelve times, rest a bit, and then continue with the next movement.

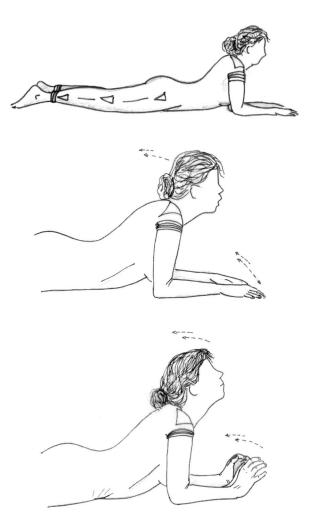

27. *Seated, Two Lateral Movements with the Head*

For the following movements, remain seated with your legs crossed in the simplest, most comfortable, and traditional way, with your fists resting on your knees and your back straight, as in the drawings. If you find this position uncomfortable, don't worry, just find a better position, on the floor, in a chair, or on your bed.

The first movements in this position work with the top third of your body: your head and neck. During each movement you must keep your eyes closed.

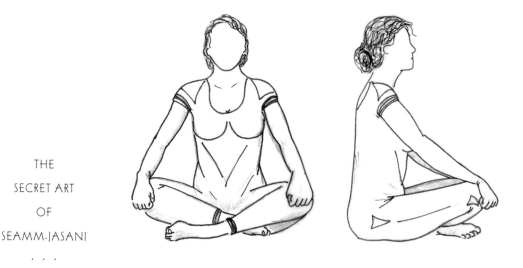

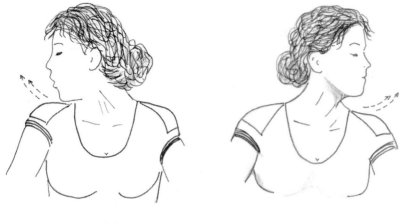

exhale   inhale

Make two short movements to each side, laterally as if shaking your head "no" in western cultures. Begin by moving your head twice to your left while inhaling twice (nnnsss . . . nnnsss . . .), then immediately to your right, exhaling twice (hhhaaa . . . hhhaaa . . .). Always inhale to one side and exhale to the other, every breath coordinated with one movement to each side. Do not pause during this exercise. Keep going, following the drawings.

When executing these movements with the top third of your body, always keep your eyes closed. This keeps you relaxed and also helps to avoid any dizziness.

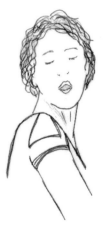

lateral view

These head movements are specially designed to release the tensions produced in the neck and shoulders, since this area collects all of the tension produced by bad posture and nervous energy.

Execute about twelve movements on each side and continue with the following movement.

. . .

28. *Front Movement, Up and Down*

Begin in the same position as in the last movement. Keep your eyes closed and your head straightened. Now make two short movements of your head up and back, inhaling twice (nnnsss . . . nnnsss . . .), then bring your chin to your chest twice, exhaling each time (hhhaaa . . . hhhaaa . . .).

Count to 12 and continue.

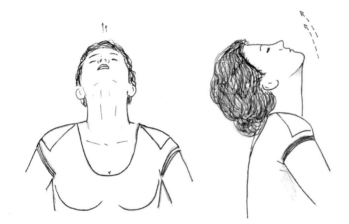

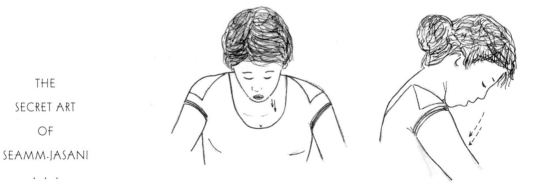

29. Circular Movement with the Head

Sit in the same position as before, but with your head relaxed and your chin down. Remember to keep your eyes closed. Now, following the drawings, turn your head clockwise while inhaling (nnnsss . . .) until you return to the beginning. Then exhale (hhhaaa . . .) while rotating your head counterclockwise.

Make twelve circles in each direction, then slowly open your eyes according to the next movement.

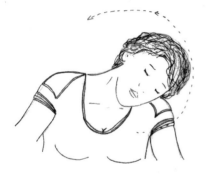
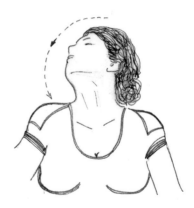
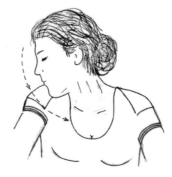

30. Visual Exercise, Blinking

Once you have finished the head movements, rest for a few seconds with your eyes closed, trying to clear your mind and enjoying this time with yourself. You will now begin to exercise your vision—work that will help to improve your internal and external sight.

After spending all of this time with your eyes closed, start blinking gently but consistently, now a bit faster, now faster and faster, slowly opening your eyes while normalizing your blinking until your eyes are completely open. This is the first tonic for your sight, providing your eyes with better lubrication and working with the orbicular muscle of the eyelid.

In the teachings of the ancient Art of mastering the mind, it is said that sight is a great window for directing and receiving energy, aside from its being the organ of our vision. The eye also controls a series of muscles that need to be stimulated in order to remain healthy and young; this exercise and the others that follow will aid in that and will help to relieve the symptoms of many different diseases of sight.

If you spend the whole day working on a computer, ignoring the warnings that your eyes give you, turn your chair around and look the other way. Try this movement and the following two, then close your eyes for a while. You will feel deep relief. Remember that we only have our two eyes and they are irreplaceable; it will take genetics and technology a long time before they will be able to replace your pair of abused eyes like a pair of old shoes.

Have you ever wondered why nowadays so many kids wear glasses? Or why professionals and students need them so often? When you have some free time, visit any poor country and you will realize that, in general, the population's sight is better. Too many good things bring bad things.

Finally, if you think that the size of this book's font is a bit too big, it is not because I was trying to make it look like it had more pages, and not because it is a children's book:

IT IS TO SPARE YOUR EYES!

NOTE: In the author's humble opinion, just as there is a warning on a pack of cigarettes alerting you to their harmful qualities, computers and books with tiny fonts should also carry a warning about the damage that they do to everyone's sight.

31. Sight Exercise, from Right to Left

For the second visual exercise, with your eyes open, put your hands on your knees or in front of you with your fingertips together in a point, as is shown in the drawings. Now, focus on the imaginary point where your fingertips come together, keeping your head centered, facing straight ahead. Then move your eyes from the point formed by one hand to the point formed by the other, continuously tracing an imaginary line from right to left, keeping your head still the whole time.

Both this and the following exercise directly stimulate the extrinsic muscles of the eyes, as well as the oblique and straight muscles surrounding them.

Count to 12, then continue.

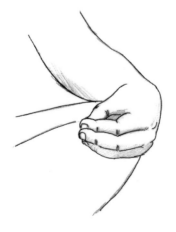

32. Sight Exercise, Up and Down

This sight exercise follows the same pattern as the last, except that in this one you put one hand up (just above eye level, pointing down) and the other hand down (pointing up), oriented on a vertical line along the center of your body. As before, do not move your head as you trace an imaginary line up and down.

Again, count to 12 and go on.

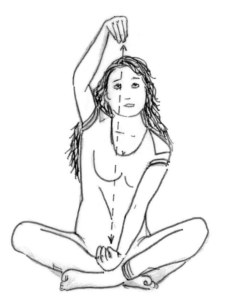

THE FIRST

THIRTY-FIVE

FUNDAMENTAL

MOVEMENTS

. . .

125

33. **Basic Hand Position**

Support your hands on your knees, loosely relaxing them as in the drawing. Now rotate your hands up, tightening them and imagining that your semistraight fingers, evenly separated one from the other (as shown in the drawings), are holding a tennis ball. Then loosen your hands and repeat the exercise in order to memorize this position.

From now on, we will call this the basic hand position.

Repeat this exercise twelve or more times, then continue.

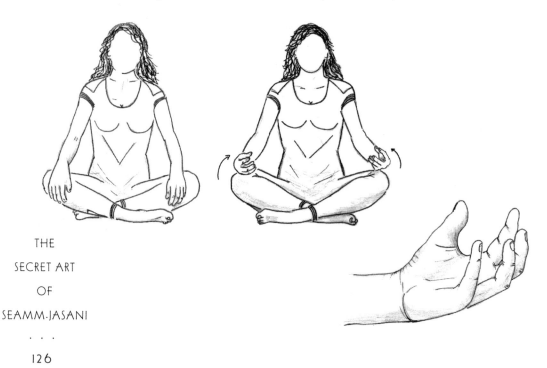

34. *Working with the Fingers*

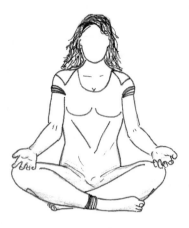

Remaining seated, you will now work with your hands and fingers. Open your hands on your knees, with your palms facing up. Now, with both hands at the same time, touch your thumb to your pinky, then to your ring finger, then to your middle finger, and finally to your index finger, one finger at a time but with a continuous and constant rhythm. The more comfortable you become with this exercise, the quicker you should try to do it.

This exercise, along with the previous one, invigorates and gives elasticity to the tendons and muscles in and around the hands, while bringing necessary heat to that bony area. If you are someone who suffers from arthritis or problems of that nature, you will find great relief by fluidly going through these movements. This last exercise will also aid your coordination.

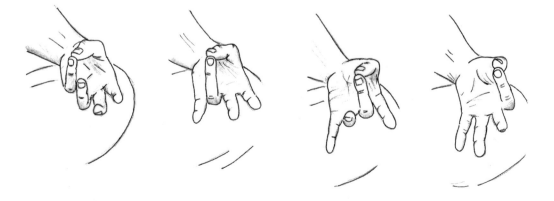

. . .

35. *Frontal Expressive Stretch*

Begin seated, with your hands at your sides, as in the drawing (remember that you can also sit in a chair or on your bed). Now, push your hands forward, inhaling deeply (nnnsss . . .). Wake up your face by making an expression that is totally serious, concentrated, almost angry! Quickly return to the initial position, exhaling (hhhaaa . . .) and loosening your expression, smiling, making your face happy and really freeing yourself!

Imagine intensely and you will be greatly relieved. Keep the serious face on for a few seconds, then by loosening your face you give yourself life! Don't follow the fashion of "developed" coun-

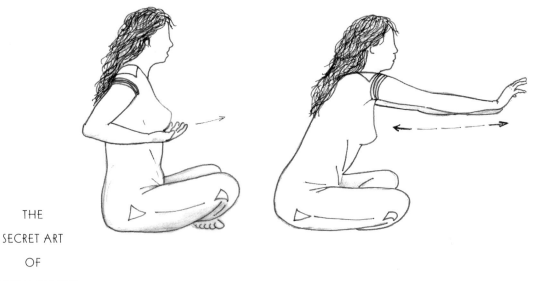

tries, where if you laugh or are expressive it seems a strange sickness. This movement is designed to liberate your expression, help-
...orld, if only for a few seconds,
...e the occipital frontal.
...velve times) and you will feel as
... shoulders!

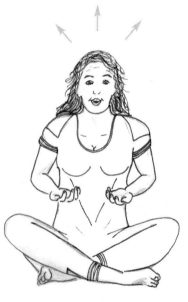

THE FIRST

THIRTY-FIVE

FUNDAMENTAL

MOVEMENTS

. . .

129

Breathing Movement of the Completion

To finish the seated movements, repeat the basic breathing technique (movement 4) in all of its details, except now you should remain sitting. Bring your hands together and, with your tongue in your palate, inhale (nnnsss . . .) as you bring your hands slowly upward in a great circle, holding the air in your lungs for a few seconds as your hands reach the top of the circle. Then lower your arms as you exhale, letting your tongue drop, rounding your lips and making the "hhhaaa . . ." sound from your throat.

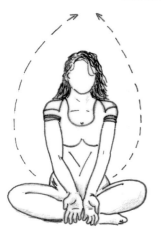

Congratulations!

With this, we have completed the "Art of Awakening." Now we are prepared, mentally and physically, to begin the coordinative movements, the fluent meditation of the Second Art.

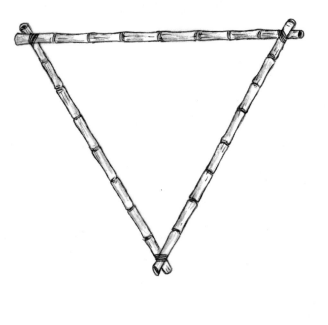

THREE STEPS FOR MEDITATION AND TWENTY MOVEMENTS OF ACTIVE RELAXATION

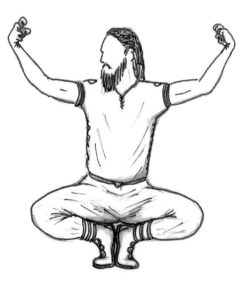

"The true art is endless, for you can never
know its entirety."

Second Art

SEAMM·JASANI
The Art for Eternal Youth

It is in this Second Art that we bring together movements that are soft and harmonious, learn coordination and breathing techniques, and begin our meditation.

Remember that the drawings are all frontal and lateral. Their order is kept consistent, so you will know which drawings are associated with which movements.

Once you have finished the final cycle of the previous Art and are standing again, relax and loosen your arms and legs a little. Now, still standing normally, repeat the basic breathing technique twice. Once you have finished this, you will be ready and warmed up, both physically and mentally, to begin this stage.

The system of movements that you are about to begin creates a chain, linking one movement to the next. You will see that from one movement is born another, more complex, until they complete a pattern that creates and defines a basic corporeal language. Follow the teacher and, with a little study, you will easily understand the movements and will be able to execute them without this book in front of you: this should be your goal.

Now, let's live the Art for Eternal Youth!

Three Steps for Meditation

Now that you have completed the First Art of movements, you are ready for a new sort of work, divided into three stages: a basic system of discipline and meditation for your mind, as well as a methodology for the execution of the movements. You can practice this system of meditation anywhere, independently; or you can add it to the rest of the exercises, as explained later in the book.

Inner Movement

Begin this meditation sitting cross-legged on the floor (First Art, movement 27, first figure). If you find this uncomfortable, don't worry, just sit or lie down comfortably.

Meditation is nothing more than a way to order, or channel, our thoughts. To view meditation as a technique to annul our thoughts, or to lead us to a state of "emptiness," as many people say, could not be farther from reality. It is simply another misunderstanding, just like the one requiring us to sacrifice and cause pain to our bodies and minds in order to become more "spiritual." These are primitive concepts, developed from a repressive mentality by a culture with sadomasochistic proclivities. This requirement of suffering, this whipping the body and flagellating the mind, are typical characteristics of chauvinist, primitive societies, and when discussing meditation and like subjects, we realize that they too have been influenced by such ignorance. I am sorry for expressing myself so bluntly, especially if by chance you have taken this personally, due to some custom, personal belief, or bad habit. I would like to write more openly on this subject but my editor, for the time being at least, is holding me in check.

Following this analysis of the mind and the development of its energy, you will see that this energy is ceaseless: it is in constant motion. If it is not one thing then it is another, but something is always making us go. In general, we tend to let ourselves follow negativity: problems, vanity, conflicts, social goals, and everything else that makes us stressed. If we try to make our minds blank, all we

THREE STEPS
FOR MEDITATION
AND TWENTY
MOVEMENTS

. . .

137

are going to do is think about the things that we don't want to think about! "Mind," said an old poet, "is a constant flow . . ." a river, or the water: it can flow, evaporate, return as a beneficent rain; it can be the sea and its waves, but it cannot stop moving. Based upon this, our work is simple, but real—to conduct our psychological energy and use it in tandem with the movements.

If you want this to be effective, you must trust entirely in your imagination; you will begin to think of imagination as meditation. So be positive and believe in your imagination; we owe to it everything creative that humanity has ever made. If not for imagination, we would still live in an era of obscurantism and ignorance, the kind that has delayed so much of our evolution as living beings. Trust in your inner energy: the great geniuses (so very few in number) did it while the rest followed negativity and mass mentality, going always by what other people say.

36. "The Feeding"

In order to make this system effective, we will begin by analyzing the Inhalation Process (described in First Art, movement 4)—specifically the internal processes: tongue in your palate, inhaling through the nose, etcetera.

During this stage of meditation, you must imagine that the air coming in through your nose is laden with an invisible energy and strength that is highly beneficial, almost dense. During the process of breathing, from the beginning of inhalation until you reach maximum capacity, you will have time to direct your thoughts, to watch (with your imagination!) the energy and strength entering your body. Give it a good taste and a pleasant smell—the breathing is much more positive when you do it on a farm, on the beach, or anywhere outside, which naturally smells much nicer. You can scent the place where you are practicing, or you can just use your imagination! At the same time, imagine that the "food" has some invisible "vitamins" that strengthen us internally, to remedy our various diseases and problems. This process will be called inhalation and "feeding" (drawing, right).

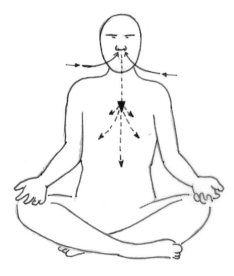

Your success in this depends on your imagination. It doesn't matter if you are a skeptical, materialistic person—it is even bet-

THREE STEPS
FOR MEDITATION
AND TWENTY
MOVEMENTS

. . .

139

ter! Think about this: if you had lived five hundred years ago, what would you have thought if someone told you that they could bring people back to life with electric shocks, or that the air is full of radio waves of different frequencies that exist even though they are invisible? Come to your own conclusions; the air is the first "food" that we consume once we are born, absorbed by its own digestive system, the lungs. Now think . . . what if the air contained other "elements" besides oxygen, nitrogen, etcetera? And what if those other "elements" could be better received and metabolized through simple mental magnetic emanation?

37. *Inner Expansion*

The second stage of our meditation is the process by which we contain and retain the air that we have just inhaled. In this period, which can last from three to eight seconds, you must channel your thoughts and imagine the food that is now inside of you being distributed to your entire body—trunk, arms, legs, head—making your whole organism glow as it is internally renewed. Everything on your inside is shining now, all expanding: every organ, bone, and muscle, and especially your mind. Use every positive thought, forget about the rest of the world (even for just a few seconds), and focus all of that positive energy on yourself, your vitality, and your perfection.

This will be called concentration and "inner expansion."

If you have some sort of disease that affects an organ or specific zone of your body, center the force of your thoughts on that organ or affected zone. You will see it heal sooner. The mind has enormous powers: if you learn how to use them positively, you will be amazed at the benefits it can give you.

When discussing the powers of the mind, someone who has seen too many movies will inevitably ask if he can hypnotize someone, or influence the decisions of others. I am afraid to disappoint the believers, but they are completely wrong. Mind is an "auto-blocking circuit" that simply rejects any unwanted information, as if it had a security guard or a jail keeper. If someone accepts a determined proposition, it is only because he or she pins interests or convenience on the proposal, be they materialistic, vain, adulatory, or escapist. Every single one of us, in different ways, is conscious of what we do, even when playing idiot when it is favorable to act in that way.

Well, I won't go further on this. Instead, I will continue with the third part of the meditation.

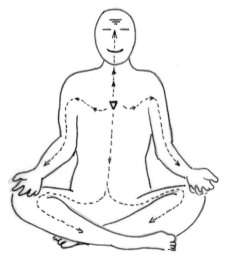

38. *Liberation*

This third stage consists of the process that accompanies the exhalation. While the air comes out through your throat, gently scratching it, imagine everything negative expelled from your body in your exhalation, the air taking it all away. Feel your body ridding itself of every disease as you throw away every pain, ache, and intolerant thought..

This will be called exhalation and "liberation."

With this system you will feel much better, fully relieved!

Imagination is a great force—trust it and trust yourself, do not repress your expansion. Use these exercises to rid yourself of negativity, to cleanse yourself and fill up with a new force, infinitely larger and more positive. In order to fully charge a battery, you must first discharge it fully, otherwise you shorten its life. The human body and mind work in a similar way.

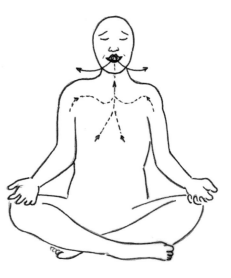

Once you have studied these three movements of meditation and after having executed them sitting up or lying down, you can add them to the different movements that you will learn and to the different forms you will see.

39. *Resting Position*

Begin this first movement by standing normally, with your arms resting in front of your body and your palms facing up, left hand over right in what we call the "resting position." All of the breathing techniques will begin from this position, as will some of the movements.

The resting position is a technique of discipline and order, as well as a sign of the balance of body and mind. Resting in it, you produce a *unified magnetic field,* which emanates forces of harmony and tranquility for you and for those who surround you. Practice it and you will see how it increases your level of concentration and your auric emanation. It is an old Seamm-Jasani trick!

The drawings show this position both frontally and laterally.

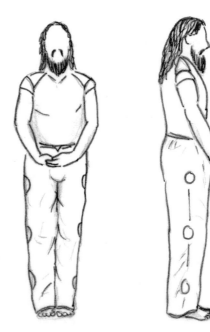

40. Normal Position

Begin from the Resting Position (movement 39). While you inhale (nnnsss . . .), bring both hands to your sides as shown in the drawing, using the basic hand position (First Art, movement 33). We will call this "Normal Position," with your arms pulled back and your hands at the level of your floating ribs.

Contain your breath for three seconds, then bring your arms back to Resting Position as you exhale (hhhaaa . . .).

When you bring your hands to your sides, your fingers should be slightly separated and facing forward. Repeat this exercise about twelve times.

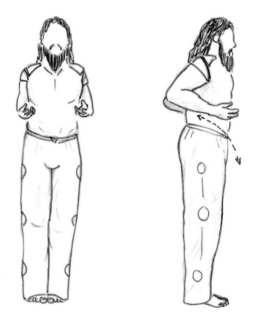

41. *Individual Projection of Energy*

Begin this movement by bringing your hands to your sides, just as in Normal Position.

Now, inhale as you bring your right hand forward. Your fingers should point forward, as if you were holding a small ball (again this is the basic hand position, First Art, movement 33). As you extend your arm, turn your hand in a circular motion—let your arm follow your hand. Look closely at the drawings: your right hand should move counterclockwise as your whole hand follows your thumb.

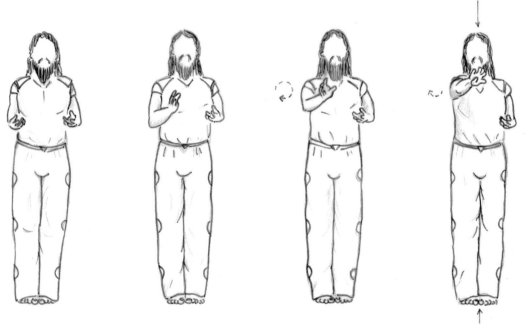

Figure 11a   Figure 11b   Figure 11c   Figure 11d

. . .

You will feel a slight tension in your hand as you turn it, and it will relax when you complete the movement.

The drawings below show the completion of the twisting motion, detailing the hand projection and the final inverse twist.

Slowly return your right arm to its initial position as you simultaneously extend your left arm, following the same form. Your left hand should turn clockwise as you extend your arm. To better understand the mechanics of this, study the next set of drawings.

In these drawings you see the same movement that we began with, but now both hands are included as they pass each other, one extending and the other retracting. Remember to inhale as you extend your right arm and to exhale as your left arm comes forward and you bring your right arm back.

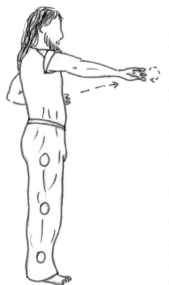

Figure 11d
(lateral)

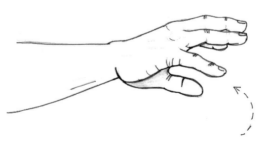

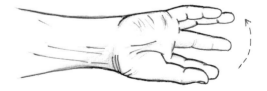

There are several important factors in developing a perfect technique:

1. Make sure to keep your back straight. The majority of back and abdominal problems come from bad positioning of your back.

2. Keep your shoulders straight, only moving your arms and not the rest of your body. When you project with this motion your shoulder remains still, concentrating the "heat" or energy of this movement solely in your arms, using that energy in the most efficient way. This might be difficult at first, but it is just part of the movement . . . you will find that with effort and time you will overcome any problems.

3. You should project so that your arm when fully extended is in front of your throat, and your hand should be centered along the midline of your body (figure 11d).

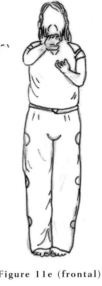
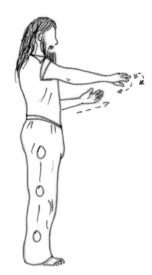

Figure 11e (frontal)   Figure 11e (lateral)

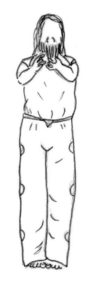
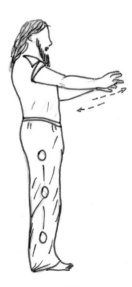

Figure 11f (frontal)   Figure 11f (lateral)

. . .

This is everything that you need in order to have a cleanly executed, precise, and harmonious technique. When you begin the movement by projecting with your right arm, use the same breathing technique that you have been using throughout, inhaling (nnnsss . . .) as you extend your right arm. The arm's gentle path should last as long as your inhalation, which, with time, will grow longer and longer. When your arm is fully extended and your wrist is twisted, hold the air in your lungs for about three seconds. Now, making good use of all of the potential energy that the movement has produced, bring back your right arm while simultaneously projecting your left, exhaling (hhhaaa . . .) for the duration of your arm's projection. Count three seconds and extend the right arm, repeating the whole movement. Remember that for both inhalation and exhalation, you should follow the same breathing technique as always—inhale through the nose, exhale through the throat.

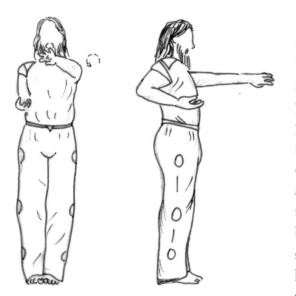

Figure 11g (frontal)   **Figure 11g (lateral)**

We have gone over this movement in minute detail because it is the base of the entire chain: it is completely normal if this movement feels strange when you are first learning it, because all of the muscles in your arm (triceps, biceps, brachial, cubital) are working rotationally. No one is accustomed to this, as there is no kind of exercise or technique, Western or Eastern, where you work your arm this way. This specific sort of exercise will benefit you greatly—it is a special tonic for your body!

Once you understand the basic technique, you can execute this movement continuously, making sure to stop a few seconds between inhalation and exhalation and vice versa. You should repeat the inhalation and exhalation cycle about twelve times, then after resting for a moment continue with your studies.

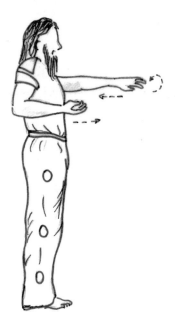

Figure 11h

42. Double Frontal Projection of Energy

For this next movement, begin with your hands in the initial position from the last movement, Normal Position. From this position, project with both arms, always keeping your shoulders straight: they do not move!

When projecting your arms forward, inhale (nnnsss . . .) until both arms are fully extended and both hands are twisted, as in the last movement. When both arms are fully extended, contain your inhalation for about three seconds, then slowly bring your arms back while exhaling harmoniously (hhhaaa . . .), following the same pattern as in the last movement, only this time with both arms. When both arms are fully extended they should be no farther apart from each other than the width of a single thumb. This movement will be called "Double Frontal Projection."

The drawings show the complete sequence.

Remember that as your arms return to your sides they must follow the same path as their extension. Execute this movement several times, resting for about three seconds between each projection.

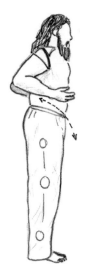
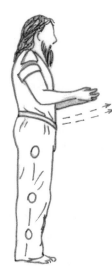
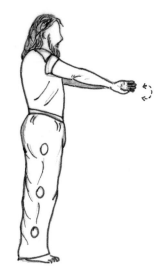

Figure 12a (lateral)   Figure 12b (lateral)   Figure 12c (lateral)

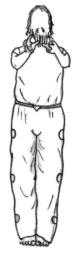

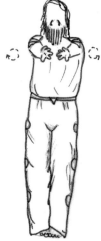

Figure 12a (frontal)   Figure 12b (frontal)   Figure 12c (frontal)

. . .

151

43. Double Lateral Projection of Energy

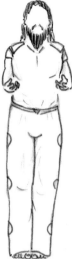

Begin this movement from the same Normal Position as before. Now, as you inhale, project both of your arms laterally, as if you were pushing two imaginary walls away from you. At your arms' fullest projection twist your wrists—just as in the previous movements. When your arms are fully extended, hold them there, containing the air in your lungs, for about three seconds, and return them, while exhaling, to Normal Position.

Rest for two or three seconds, then repeat the movement.

This movement is called "Double Lateral Projection," and you should repeat it the same number of times as the others.

Figure 13a

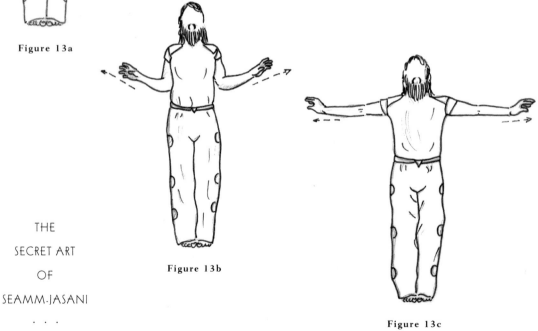

Figure 13b

Figure 13c

44. *Frontal High Double Projection of Energy*

Begin again in Normal Position. Now, extend both arms to the front as you inhale, twisting your wrists as usual and keeping your hands separated by the width of only one thumb, this time not just extending your arms but raising them as well, to eye level. When both arms are extended, bend your wrists down, so the fingers are pointing at a wall in front of you—this works the muscles in your arms and back more deeply than they are used to.

This movement is called "High Double Projection," and its general mechanics are the same as those in movement 41.

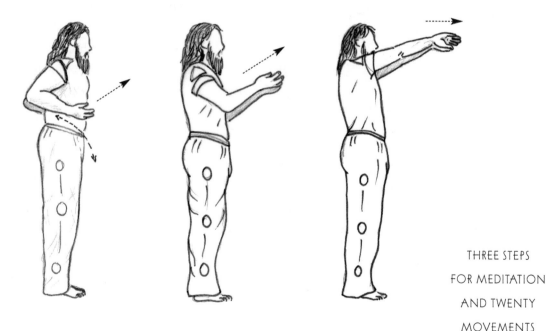

45. *Universal Position*

Now we will begin some basic movements for your entire body, beginning with the simplest and becoming more complex, until you are able to execute what we call a complete "form."

Begin this movement again in Normal Position, but with your feet together and your back totally straight. Begin by turning your left foot diagonally (45 degrees—figure 14a). Now lift your right leg as shown in figure 14b, with your toes flexed back and your foot in front of your other leg, the bottom of your raised foot parallel to the wall. Inhale (nnnsss . . .) as you are lifting your leg, then contain your breath for a few seconds as you hold your leg there. Now, slowly bring your right foot down (as if you were landing an airplane!) and open it to the right side until it rests about three feet from your left foot. For the last third of its "journey," both opening and returning, your foot must drag on the floor.

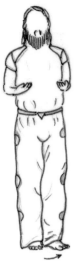

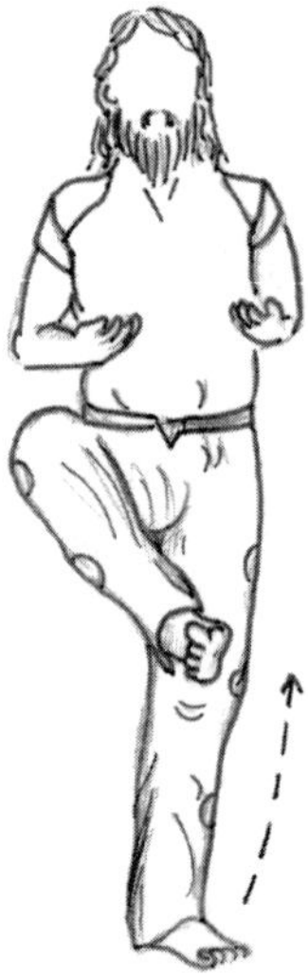

Figure 14a
(frontal)

Figure 14b
(frontal)

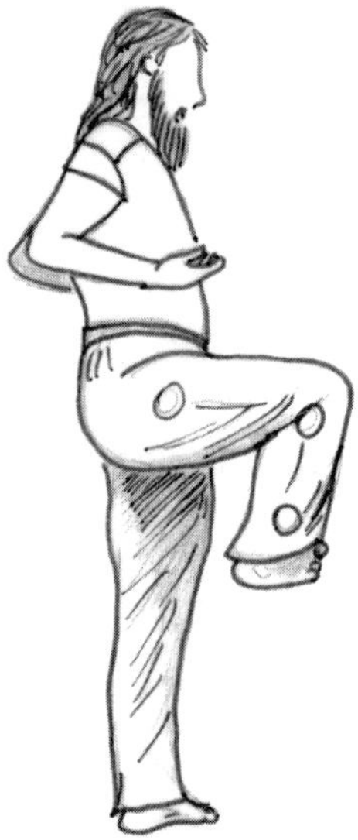

Figure 14b
(lateral)

The entirety of the opening movement, from the point where your foot is raised until it stops on the floor, is accompanied by an exhalation (hhhaaa . . .). When you finish exhaling, your body should remain straight as your legs create a gentle arch, your knees slightly bent.

It is not necessary to open your legs exactly three feet, nor is it necessary to bend your legs severely: look only for what is comfortable for your body and your initial ability. The same is true when lifting your leg: do what you feel comfortable doing and no more. An alternative, shorter, position is shown on page 156.

This movement will be called "Universal Position."

To return to your initial position, begin by lifting your right foot gently, inhaling (nnnsss . . .) as you follow an arc over and up, until your foot is in front of the other knee, parallel to the wall. Now as you bring your foot back down, exhale (hhhaaa . . .) and put your feet together again. Finish by closing your left foot, the opposite of how you began. I have added a small drawing that describes the pattern of both feet.

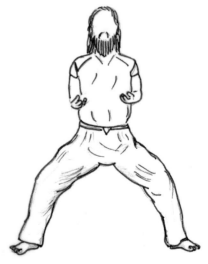

Figure 14c
(frontal)

Universal Position

This position will make your calf, thigh, and buttocks stronger while also cultivating your balance
and fluidity.

Execute this movement five or so times. You
should also practice it on the other side, as this will
be useful later on.

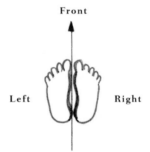

Front

Left   **Right**

Normal Position

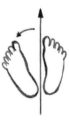

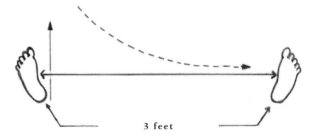

3 feet

alternate position

46. *Individual Position and Projection*

This series of movements combines all of the basic patterns that you have learned so far. Begin by executing the previous movement, closing and then opening again, but the second time do not close your feet—remain standing in Universal Position, as still as you can be.

Without moving the rest of your body, use all of your concentration to extend your arms just as in movement 41, the Individual Projection of Energy. Inhale as you extend your right arm, contain the air in your lungs, then exhale as you project with your left arm. Concentrate on the fluidity and fluency of the movement as you repeat it about eight times.

When you are done bring both arms to your sides and close the position exactly as described in movement 45.

This is a very complete exercise for both upper and lower body.

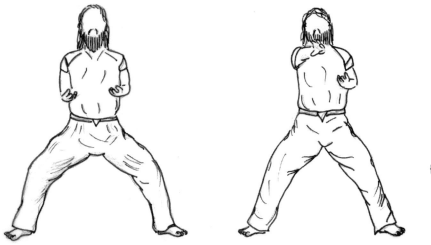

THREE STEPS
FOR MEDITATION
AND TWENTY
MOVEMENTS

. . .

157

47. *Double Frontal Position and Projection*

Again execute movement 45 twice, the second time remaining in Universal Position. Now execute movement 42, Double Frontal Projection, extending both arms to the front as you inhale, and exhaling as you return. Keep in mind the fluency of your movement, its technical precision, and the strength in your hands. When fully extended, hold the air in your lungs for a few seconds before returning slowly. When your arms return, wait a few seconds before beginning the movement again.

Forget the tiredness that you feel in your legs—conduct your mind, do not let it rule over you. Concentrate only on your arms and the energy that they produce as you repeat the movement about eight times, keeping your legs completely still.

After resting for a few seconds, you are ready for the next movement.

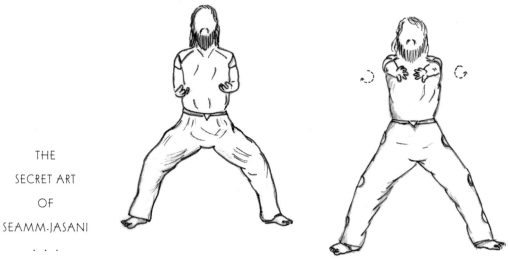

48. Double Circular Position and Projection of Energy

Repeat Universal Position as before, but this time you will execute a new movement, called Double Circular Projection.

Begin by bringing your arms in front of your torso, as the drawing shows, without stretching or straining them. Simply imagine that you are holding a ball in front of you. Now twist your hands to the front, projecting with your palms and keeping your fingers behind them, out of

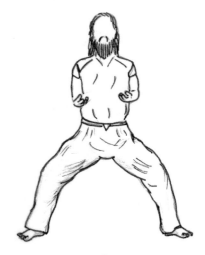

Universal Position
Figure 15a

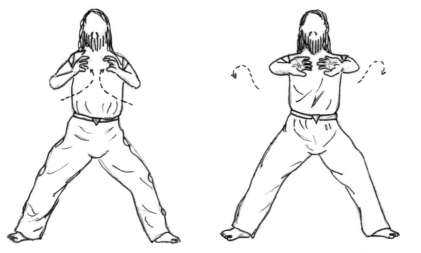

Figure 15b (frontal)

Figure 15c (frontal)

THREE STEPS
FOR MEDITATION
AND TWENTY
MOVEMENTS

. . .

159

the way. When fully extended, your arms should form a semicircle in front of your chest, as shown in the drawings.

Inhale while you are projecting and exhale while returning your arms to their normal position.

Execute this movement eight to twelve times.

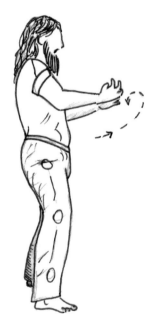

Figure 15b (lateral)

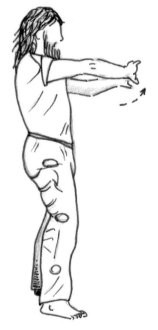

Figure 15c (lateral)

49. Form 1: Dawn

So far, we have completed one basic stage, learning arm movements and Universal Position, then joining them.

You are now ready to learn and execute two complete forms: a simpler one and a more complex one, both of which include breathing, steps, coordination, movements, fluidity, and basic meditation.

On this, the forty-ninth movement, you will learn Form 1, called "Dawn" because its movements extend just as the morning sun.

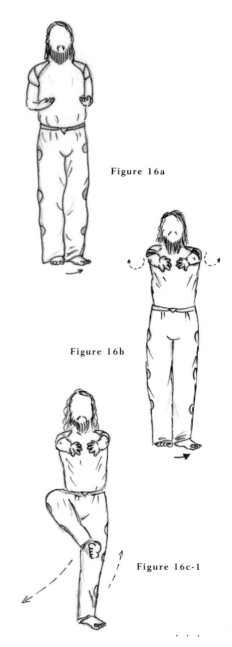

Figure 16a

Figure 16b

Figure 16c-1

a. Initial Position. Begin in Resting Position (movement 39), then change to Normal Position while opening your foot diagonally.

b. Double Frontal Projection. Inhale as you extend both of your arms forward.

c. Universal Position. Lift your right foot and open to Universal Position as you exhale. Keep both of your arms extended (do not move them!).

d. Now, bring your arms back to Normal Position, as you inhale.

. . .

e. Double Lateral Projection. Exhale as you extend your arms to your sides, as in movement 42.

Now, go through the same movements, but this time closing the form:

f. Inhale as you return your arms to Normal Position. Your legs are still in Universal Position.

g. Double Frontal Projection. Extend both of your arms forward as you exhale. Hold your arms in that position.

h. Now, twisting your right foot so that it faces front again, gently close Universal Position as you inhale, bringing your right leg back so that it stands next to the left. Keep your arms in front of you!

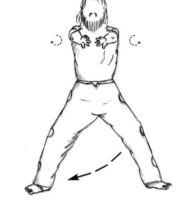

Figure 16c-2
complete position

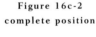

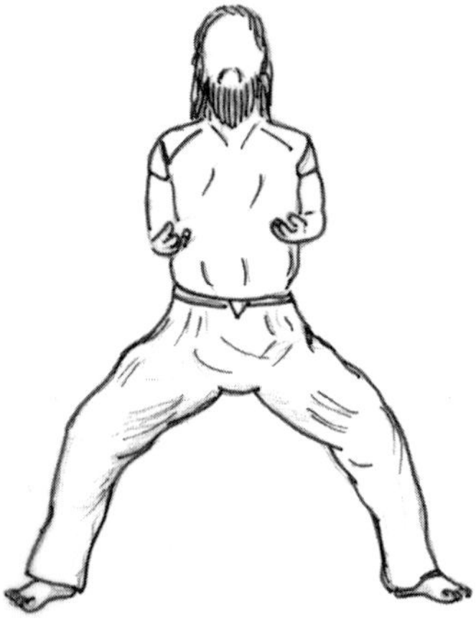

Figure 16d

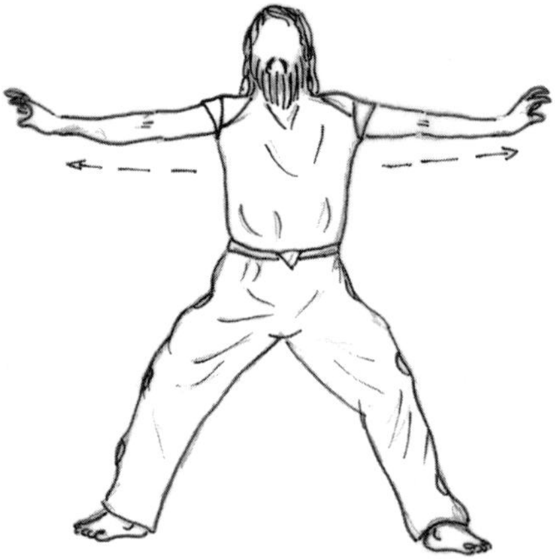

Figure 16e

i.   To complete the form, exhale as you now bring your arms back to your sides, returning to Normal Position before lowering your hands to resting position.

You have returned to the beginning, and in this way have completed Form 1, "Dawn."

This form summarizes and tests your balance and solidity, your fluency with the movements, and your command over the breathing techniques—an excellent exercise for relaxation and vitality! Practice this form often and you will see as it helps you through all of your pains and obligations. For our course, repeat Form 1 three times before going on to the next movement.

You will feel like a new person!

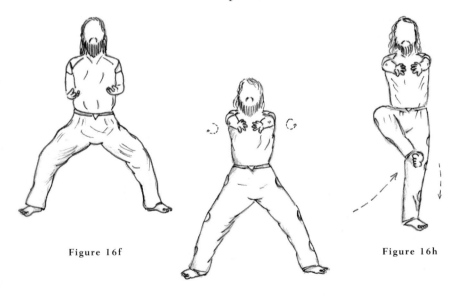

Figure 16f

Figure 16g

Figure 16h

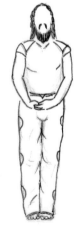

Figure 16i

· · ·

50. Form 2: Awakening

This next Form is a little bit more complicated, as you have to use the three techniques of meditation in order to make it complete. Just like cooking, bit by bit we are gathering new ingredients, positive energies, and a steady hand, so the result will always be excellent!

a.   Initial Position. Begin from Resting Position, then bring your hands to Normal Position as you open your left foot diagonally. Inhale, using your imagination as in the meditation techniques, imagining that your are "feeding" on the air as you execute Double Frontal Projection. Contain the air in your lungs as you imagine the energy flowing through your body, the "expansion" explained in movement 37.

b.   Lift your right foot and open to Universal Position, exhaling, imagining that you are releasing all of the negative energy through your exhalation. Remember to keep your arms extended!

c.   Inhale ("feeding"), bringing your arms to Normal Position. Contain the air for a few seconds as you imagine the energy coursing through your body.

d.   Now, exhale ("liberation") as you execute Double Lateral Projection, using all of your strength to slowly push the two laterally advancing walls away from you.

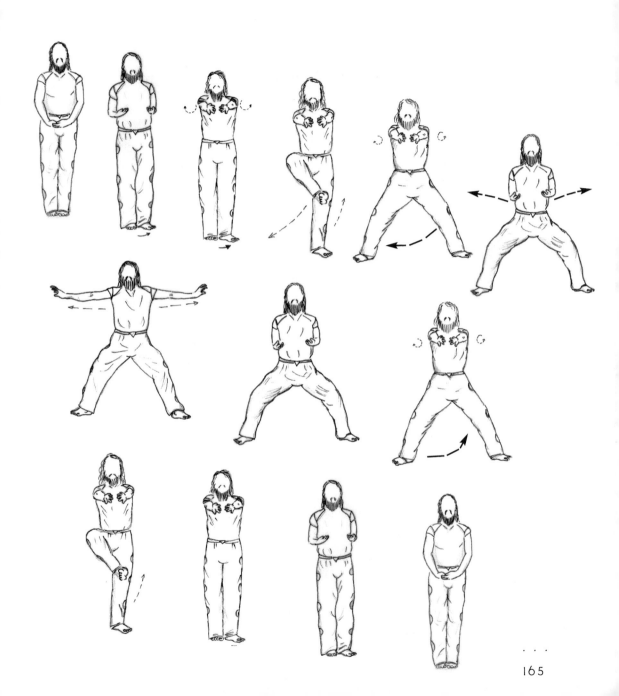

165

e.   Bring your arms back as you inhale ("feeding"), to Normal Position. Again, contain the air in your lungs as you "expand," again.

f.   Extend both of your arms forward, exhaling while you "free yourself."

g.   Now inhale as you close Universal Position, feeding slowly on the air. Begin by twisting your right foot, lifting it, and placing it next to your left foot. Your arms remain extended.

h.   Now exhale, ridding yourself of all negativity, as you bring your arms first to Normal Position, then lowering them to Resting Position.

You can begin this form by opening to the other side as well, following the same pattern of movements. It is not as easy as you think!

If you dedicate a little bit of time to this form, you will see your achievements grow huge!

51. *Right Basic Step*

You will now learn a new kind of movement—we will call it a "Basic Step." This movement teaches you how to move harmoniously, with elegance, while simultaneously improving your balance and giving necessary energy to your body's lower third as you learn how to control and make your legs, feet, and hips stronger. Don't worry if you can't instantaneously control this process; with a little dedication, you will have no problem at all!

The Basic Step is made up of these movements:

a. Begin with both of your feet together as you stand in Normal Position. Keep your hands in Normal Position through this whole movement, giving your entire concentration to the step itself.

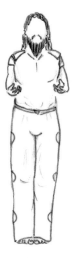

Figure 17a

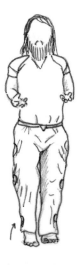

Figure 17b
(frontal)

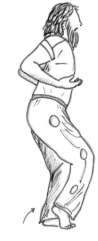

Figure 17b
(lateral)

THREE STEPS
FOR MEDITATION
AND TWENTY
MOVEMENTS

. . .

167

b. Flex both of your knees. Without moving the front of your foot, lift your right heel off the ground.

c. Inhale as you lift your right foot, keeping your toes flexed back.

d. Exhale as you lower your foot, moving it back and to the right. Your foot should trace a semicircle, first backward and then to the right, until it comes gliding to rest behind you and to your right. Make sure to look at the illustrations and make a note of this position—it is a starting point, and you will come back to it.

e. Rest your foot on the floor, as in the drawings. Your feet should be parallel to each other, pointing forward.

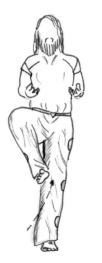 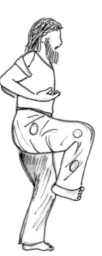 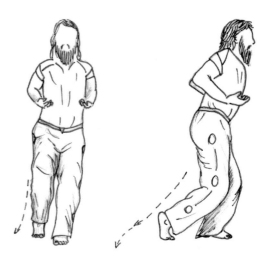

Figure 17c (frontal)   Figure 17c
(lateral)

Figure 17d
(frontal and lateral)

. . .

Now you are ready to step forward.

f. Inhaling, return almost to Normal Position, your foot following the same path back, until you are again holding it in front of your knee (as in figure 17c). Instead of returning your foot to the floor where it began, exhale as you bring your right foot forward, again tracing a gentle arc until it lands softly, in front of you and to the right. Now you have completed a semicircle, a whole forward step on your right side. Make sure to study the drawings carefully.

g. Now it is time to step back, which is a bit more complicated. You should follow the same path by which you advanced, but in reverse. Follow the drawings. Begin by flexing your left leg a little to compensate for your weight. Now, lift your right

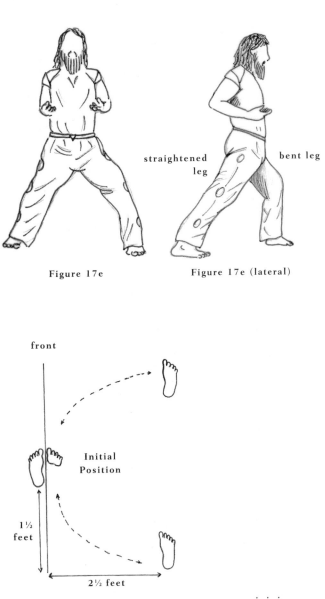

straightened leg

bent leg

Figure 17e

Figure 17e (lateral)

front

Initial Position

1½ feet

2½ feet

foot slowly, bringing it back over the same arc as before. Inhale through this movement, until your right foot is in front of your left knee, without putting it on the floor.

h. Now exhale as you bring your leg back and to the right, tracing the same curve as when you first moved it, and finishing in that same place—you are back to the first position of the movement!

i. From here you can repeat the entire movement three or four times in order to gain a better command of its mechanics and balance. You do not need to imitate the illustrations exactly; what is important is that you do your best and feel comfortable with what you are doing. In a short amount of time you will find yourself improving drastically.

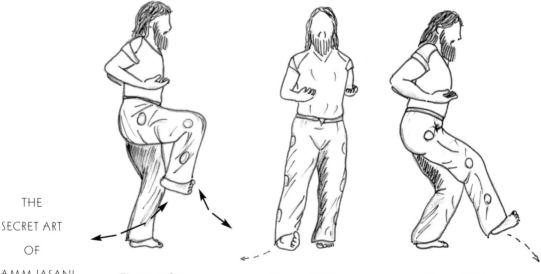

Figure 17f-1   Figure 17f-2
                               (frontal)

Figure 17f-2
(lateral)

After you have practiced this movement a few times, inhale as you lift your right foot and bring it to the starting point (raised and next to your other leg). Now exhale as you return to Resting Position.

This is a fundamental step, and it is excellent for improving your sense of balance and space along with your concentration, physical confidence, and grace in movement. I won't go into tedious detail about which particular leg muscles you are working, because you are working with all of them: gluteus, medium abductor, sartorius, etcetera. If you work slowly and technically, you will find yourself sweating a lot—this movement may look simple, like a cat's silent walk, but you will find it much more rigorous than you expect! In the old traditions of this Art, it is said that whoever masters these steps will follow the "law of silence"; they will be able to walk or run without being heard, remaining unnoticed where the rest is obvious.

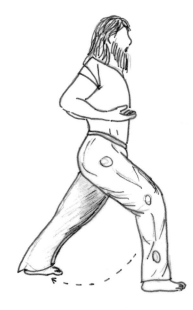

Figure 17f-3
final position

THREE STEPS
FOR MEDITATION
AND TWENTY
MOVEMENTS

. . .

171

52. Left Basic Step

This movement is identical to the last, except that it is on the opposite side—with your left leg.

a.   Begin with both of your feet together as you stand in Normal Position. Keep your hands in Normal Position throughout this whole movement, giving your entire concentration to the step itself.

b.   Flex both of your knees. Lift your left heel off the ground.

c.   Inhale as you lift your left foot, keeping your toes pointed backward.

d.   Exhale as you lower your foot, moving it back and to the left. Your foot should trace a semicircle, first backward and then to the left, until it comes gliding to rest.

e.   Put your foot on the floor, as in the drawing on page 173. Your feet should be parallel to each other, pointing forward.

Now you are ready to step forward.

f.   Inhaling, return to Normal Position, your foot following the same path back, until you are again holding it in front of your knee (as in figure 17c). Instead of returning your foot to the floor where it began, exhale as you bring your left foot forward, again tracing a gentle arc until it lands softly in front of you and to the left. Now you have completed a semicircle, a whole forward step on your left side.

g.   Now it is time to step back, which is a bit more complicated. You should follow the same path by which you advanced, but in reverse. Follow the drawing at the right. Begin by flexing your right leg a little, to compensate for your weight. Now, lift your left foot slowly, bringing it back over the same arc as before. Inhale through this movement, until your left foot is in front of your right knee, without putting your foot on the floor.

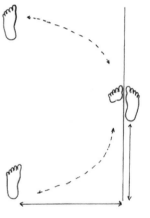

h.   Now exhale as you bring your leg back and to the left, tracing the same curve as when you first moved it, finishing in the same position.

i.   Again, repeat this movement three or four times, as practice, in order to improve your balance and strength. When you are done, lift your left foot and, inhaling, trace an arc until your feet are together again. Now exhale as you go from normal position to resting position.

NOTE: If you wish, you can combine the Right Basic Step and the Left Basic Step to walk forward, covering four or five semicircles before returning in the same way. The more you do them the more the steps will require of you, and you will spend a lot more energy (as you gain many benefits)! But, of course, it is enough at this basic stage for you to more simply review these movements.

53. Basic Step and Individual Projection

Now you have reached a level where you are ready to combine movements with these basic steps. The first movement of this sort will combine the Steps with Individual Projection (movement 41).

a.   Begin with parts a through e of the Basic Step (movement 51).

b.   When in that position, project your left arm, inhaling.

c.   Advance, keeping your left arm steady and centered in front of you. To advance, follow the movements as you have learned them in movement 51, but this time exhale for the entire duration of your advance—the whole semicircle—until your right foot comes to rest in front of you.

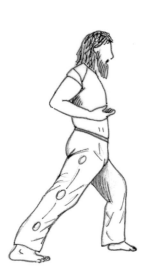

Figure 18a

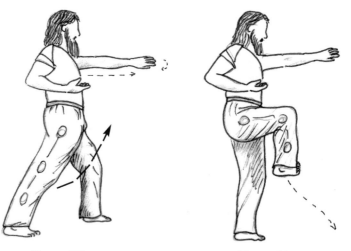

Figure 18b

Figure 18c

d.   Now, inhaling, project your right arm while bringing your left to your side.

e.   Step backward with your right foot, returning as you exhale, following the pattern set out in parts g and h of movement 51.

f.   When back in your original position, project the left hand and bring the right one to your side while inhaling. Now repeat the whole pattern three or more times, forward and backward. When you are ready to close the movement, instead of projecting again with your left arm simply bring your right arm to your side as you inhale, then exhale as you bring your right foot forward until it is next to your left, returning to Normal Position, both feet together.

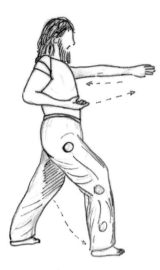

Figure 18d-1

If you would like to complicate this movement, try it on the left side, switching everything (including which arm you project).

This movement serves as the basis for all of the movements that follow; therefore, you must pay close attention to it. If you do not feel that you have properly learned it, then do not go further—it would be like painting on something before cleaning it. Be patient; study and practice this movement at your own pace, until you feel confident in its execution.

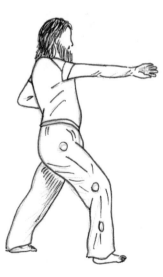

Figure 18d-2

54. Basic Step and Double Frontal Projection

Now we will combine the Basic Steps with the Double Frontal Projection.

a.   Begin with parts a through e from movement 51, Right Basic Step.

b.   Once you are in position, project both arms to the front, inhaling.

c.   Now move forward. You must combine the forward step from movement 51, exhaling the whole time, while bringing your arms in to your sides. As you step forward, exhale and bring your arms in—the exhalation should finish when your arms come to a rest at your sides, which should happen just as your foot comes to a rest in front of you.

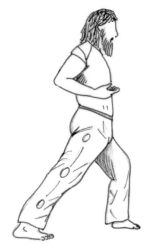

Figure 19a

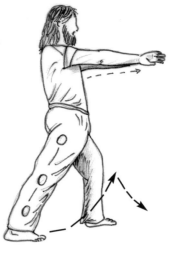

Figure 19b

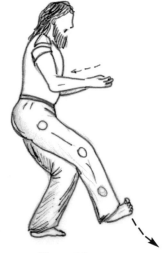

Figure 19c

d.   Again, project with both arms as you inhale.

e.   Now step backward, exhaling as you bring both arms back to your sides.

f.   Back in the original position, you should repeat this pattern three or more times. In order to close the whole movement, just follow the instructions in movement 51.

Again, if you are ambitious, you can complicate this movement by trying it on the left side.

Execute this movement patiently and quietly, following the details, and you will begin to see and feel your own magnetism. Practice this movement with *art,* elegance, imagination, and feeling, and you will improve quickly; if you like, use your imagination and the meditation techniques to enrich this movement as you activate your mind and channel its energy.

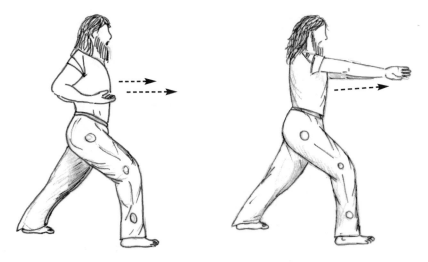

Figure 19d-1   **Figure 19d-2**

THREE STEPS

FOR MEDITATION

AND TWENTY

MOVEMENTS

. . .

177

55. *Basic Step and Double Circular Projection*

In this movement, we join the Double Circular Projection with the Basic Step.

a.   Again, begin with parts a through e from movement 51.

b.   Now that you are in position, project both arms in Double Circular Projection (movement 48), as you inhale.

c.   Now advance. As before, step forward as in movement 51, but exhaling through the whole movement. And as in the previous movement, bring both arms to your sides as you exhale and advance. Your arms should reach normal position just as your foot touches the ground.

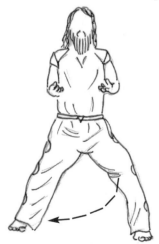

Figure 20a

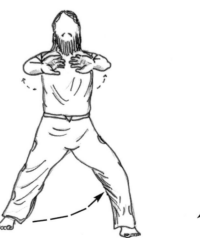

Figure 20b

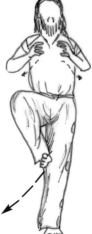

Figure 20c-1

· · ·

178

d. Project both of your arms again as you inhale.

e. Step backward as you exhale, bringing your arms back to Normal Position.

Repeat the pattern three or four times, then close the movement as before.

You can also complicate this movement by trying it out on the left side.

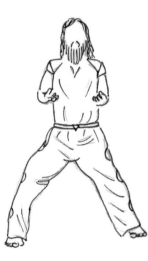

Figure 20c-2

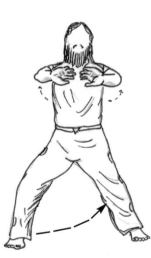

Figure 20d

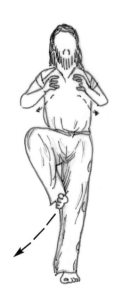

Figure 20e

56. Basic Step and Double Lateral Projection

Finally, we will combine the Basic Step with the Double Lateral Projection, to finish this cycle and prepare ourselves for Form 3.

    a.   Begin with parts a though e from movement 51.

    b.   Once in position, inhale while you project both arms to your sides, as in movement 43.

    c.   Move forward, exhaling as you advance with your leg, bringing both arms in to your sides. Your hands should reach normal position just as your foot touches the ground.

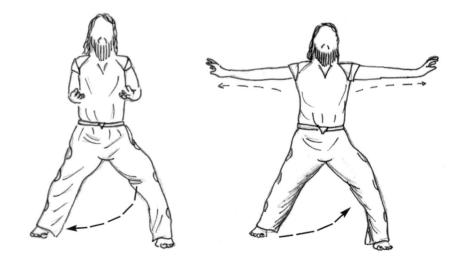

Figure 21a   Figure 21b

d.   Again, project both of your arms laterally as you inhale.

e.   Now step backward, exhaling and bringing both arms to Normal Position.

Repeat the movements three or four times, then close as in movement 51. Also as before, you can try this movement on the left side.

With just a little time, you have gained a lot of skill in the mechanics of these movements, and you are ready to learn the final form, which gathers up everything you have learned so far into a general pattern of movement.

You have already begun to learn the ancient Art for Eternal Youth—from here onward, only practice and your will can perfect it.

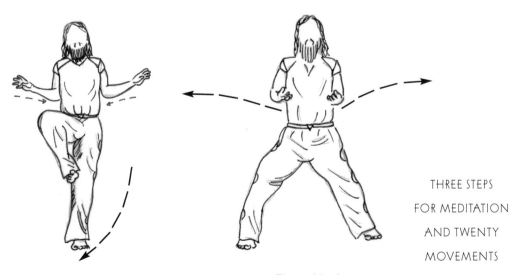

Figure 21c-1   Figure 21c-2

57. Form 3: "Union"

To complete our introductory class in this Art for Eternal Youth, we will learn and cultivate the third, or "Union," form. To understand this form, it is vital that you have command of the previous movements and forms, for the "Union" form is like putting together the pieces of a puzzle—if you have all of the pieces, it should be easy and natural. On the other hand, if you have not been a good student, you will see it immediately because you won't understand the form. Just take it slowly and do not worry—if you don't understand it, just review the movements from this stage.

Do what you understand and, without noticing it, you will discover the mechanics of what you had not understood before. The mind is overly pampered and introverted; if you push it, it closes

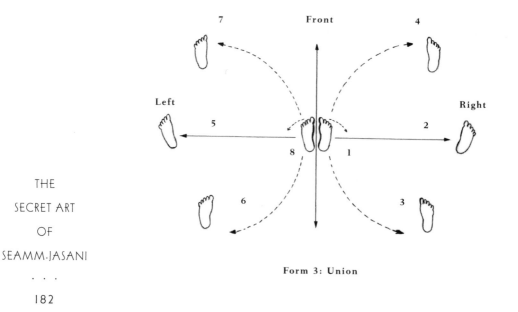

Form 3: Union

every circuit and fails to give its all. You must distract it, be kind to it; if you do this your mind will open up and it will tell you many of its secrets. Now relax and study the form of Union.

It is a good idea to learn this form first without the inhalation and exhalation, so you can memorize the movements before complicating them with the breathing and meditation techniques. Make sure to study the drawings below and on the following pages: they show all of the movements in sequence.

a.   Begin standing, in Resting Position. Now lower your arms and execute the Breathing Technique of the Great Circle. When you have completed it, bring your hands to your sides in Normal Position.

b.   Now you are ready to continue. To your right, execute Form 1 (movement 49): Double Frontal Projection (inhale), open to the right side (exhale), bring your hands to Normal Position (inhale), Double Lateral Projection (ex-

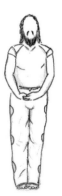 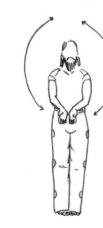 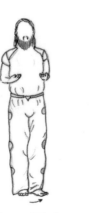 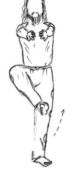

Figure 22a   Figure 22b-1

. . .

hale), bring your hands to Normal Position (inhale), then double Frontal Projection again (exhale).

c. From there, bring your right foot in as you inhale, but do not put your feet together; instead move backward with the Basic Step as you exhale and bring your arms in to Normal Position.

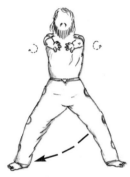 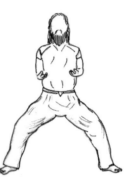 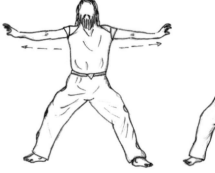

Figure 22b-2

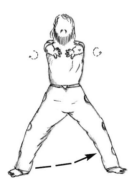 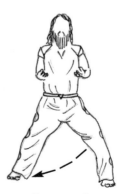 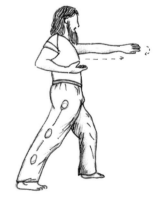

Figure 22c   **Figure 22d**

d.   Left Individual Projection, inhaling. Advance with the Right Basic Step as you exhale. Keep your arm extended.

e.   Inhale as you project your right arm. Now bring your foot back as you exhale, but, instead of bringing your foot behind you, put your feet together as you bring your right arm to your side. Now you should be in Normal Position, with your feet together.

f.   Again execute Form 1, but this time to the left side: Double Frontal Projection (inhale), open to the left side (exhale), bring your arms to Normal Position (inhale), Double Lateral Projection (exhale), bring your hands back to Normal Position (inhale), then Double Frontal Projection (exhale).

g.   From there, bring your left foot back to the right as you inhale, but do not put it down; continue moving it back-

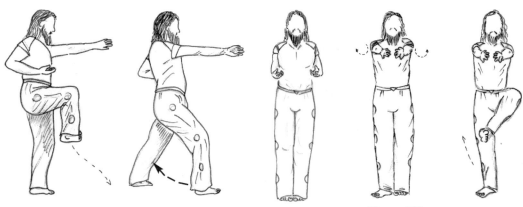

Figure 22e   Figure 22f

. . .

185

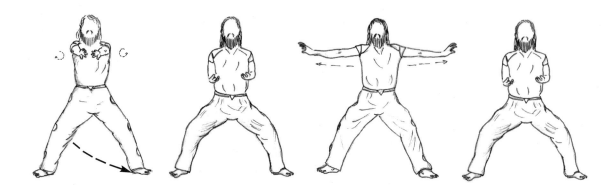

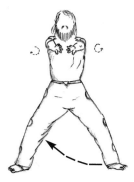

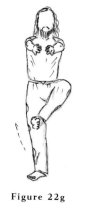

Figure 22g

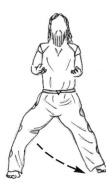

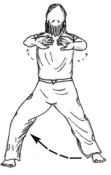

Figure 22h

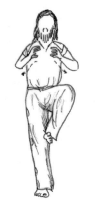

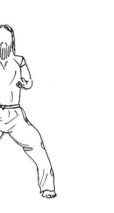

(lateral view)

ward as you exhale, just as in the Left Basic Step. Remember to bring your arms to your sides as you exhale.

h.   Double Circular Projection to the front as you inhale. Advance with the Left Basic Step, simultaneously bringing your arms in to Normal Position as you are exhaling. Now you are standing forward, with both arms at your sides.

i.   Frontal High Double Projection as you inhale. Bring your foot back as you exhale, but do not go all the way back: go only halfway, so your feet are back together. Bring in your arms as you exhale. Now you are in Normal Position, where you began.

j.   From there, lower your arms again and execute the Breathing Technique of the Great Circle, and when your arms come back down put them in Resting Position.

With all of this, you have returned to the beginning and you have begun to close the circle.

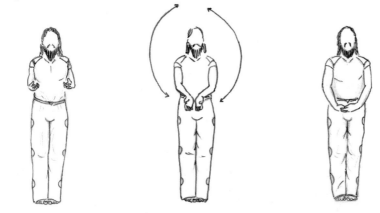

Figure 22i–j

THREE STEPS
FOR MEDITATION
AND TWENTY
MOVEMENTS

. . .

187

58. *Closing the Circle*

To finish your physical-psychical work, sit down in the Basic Position, or in any position that is more comfortable for you, so that we may finish with a movement of relaxation and vibration through sound. As you sit join your hands in your lap, then inhale deeply as you bring them up in the Breathing Technique of the Great Circle. Contain the air, then exhale gently as you lower your hands. Repeat this, inhaling again as you raise you hands, contain the air, and exhale gently but with a quieter sound in your throat, "hhhaaa . . .", until, when you are just about to finish a new sound is born, a soft "mmmmm . . ." that resounds inside of you with a fine internal vibration. When you have finished, close your eyes.

Rest your arms on your knees, sitting still with your eyes closed and relax, feeling much better after everything you have just done. You can see how this gentle sound surrounds you, leaving you quiet and clear.

Now, open your eyes: you are relieved, having dedicated some time to yourself, feeding yourself with the enormous magnetism and strength that surrounds you . . . you are ready to begin anything. Most important, you are ready to begin living happily, full of energy and imagination, learning the vastness of life all around you.

Congratulations! Congratulations!
Congratulations!
and
May the Cosmic Wind
Always Blow in Your Favor!

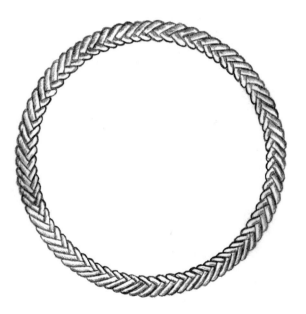

CONCLUSION

. . . The sun was already shining with its best energies, but without any unpleasantness: it seemed as if the Earth and all the living beings had arisen again in their plenitude. The morning's lesson for the beginners was just finishing; they had made many movements and were sweating profusely as more than one carried his or her own curious, personal cloud, formed by evaporating sweat. The class was closing the cycle of awakening, finishing with the same sound with which it had begun.

Once they were dismissed, they spoke happily of their new achievements and of the new movements they had been taught. Some talked about the great feeling they found in the Art, the sensation of energy and concentration, of tiredness and at the same

. . .

time renewal and strengthening, of how strange it was that after working so intensely, both physically and mentally, they felt so good, ready to do so many things, to listen, to value, and to learn.

The restless apprentice continued reviewing his movements for a few moments, a small distance from the others. Some of his movements were delicate, others strong; he expressed himself with his hands, his legs, his torso, and his face, making strange sounds, singing like some different creature. He did not want to lose what he had just learned, wanting to keep it by repeating all of the movements and gestures, making them a part of him, of his essence, until they were natural, as if he were born with them in him already. He stopped for a moment, seeming to think about something. Perhaps his mind was still on someday teaching others what he had learned. Perhaps he was thinking of how positive his "project" could be.

The guide was watching him from a distance and knew what the apprentice wanted. The guide spoke to him, almost whispering . . .

"You have bad intentions."

"Why?" asked the apprentice, again pausing in his concentrated review.

"You are still thinking of teaching the whole world . . . the world is thankless," said the guide.

"Well . . ."

"You are a black sheep," added the guide, almost smiling.

"So . . . what should I do?" the student asked.

"Life is wise, and it demands what is necessary from us. When the moment comes, you will find out . . ."

It is already dusk . . .

the mountains close their eyes

and in the distance

those who do not wish to see are left behind,

forgotten, while the emptiness

patiently distresses them.

In the Valleys of the Tides,

the sacred vestements rest

and are guarded;

the shapeless force prepares for its departure.

Have you ever felt the chafing of the wind?

Have you ever appreciated

the smile of the Universe?

Have you ever smelled

the tender flowers of the Path?

As it is . . .

. . . already it walks, it learns, it listens;

and now it travels . . .

Comments of Some Students

For thousands of years, this science has been silently passed from one generation to the next, until now. All those who have studied it have benefited from this Art and its system of movements as exercise, for overcoming disease, for inner growth, and for the discovery of the great vitality that everyone holds inside of themselves.

As a reference, we have included comments from some of the thousands of students who have in recent years studied this Art in South and North America. They have studied as private students and through various courses and workshops organized in different cities, universities, and corporations, and all have been taught by teachers trained to teach the Art of Seamm-Jasani.

Our thanks go out to all of the students and former students for their constant support and dedication, for it is always the students that make up the basis and vitality of any school.

. . .

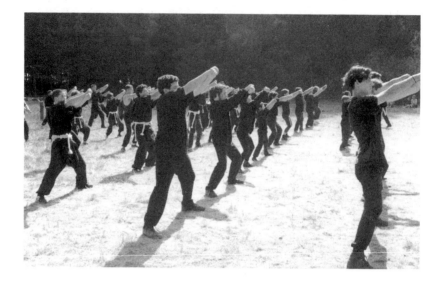

NOWADAYS it is not so often discussed that physical exercise liberates endorphins, substances within our bodies that counteract pain and stagnation throughout the body. Discouragement, sadness, and depression are internal catalysts not only of organic malfunctions (headaches, muscular pains, gastritis) but also of more serious ailments such as ulcers and cancer; thus we should not be surprised that states of happiness, comfort, and enthusiasm have real healing powers over old, chronic ailments that students often bring when they first arrive, causing them to vanish after a while. . . . Our bodies, even the weakest and most underdeveloped we have seen, are full of potentialities that one may never finish discovering and are able, with practice, to coordinate themselves in ways we believed impossible.

This can be seen in the earliest classes, as you see your problems and preoccupations left behind. This Art achieves, from a holistic point of view, to reverse the de-emphasis on man by the sciences, for man has been removed from the center of the universe by astronomical sciences, from the top of the animal kingdom by biological sciences, and from himself by psychological sciences . . .

The Seamm-Jasani, with its exercises and coordinations whose origins are lost in the depths of time, in remote places, part of a greater whole . . . centers again man on himself, takes him out of his exterior world, and develops a special sort of body-mind relation, simply called "meditation in motion."

When your body becomes elastic, reflective, serene; when your personal image is different from the one you recall; when you begin to perceive all of these changes within yourself . . . you will recall these simple words and know that the time you have devoted to the Art for Eternal Youth has not been in vain.

Sebastián Alarcón, MD,
surgeon, Uruguay
Postgraduate in anaesthesiology
specialist in clinical hypnosis

SINCE beginning my study of this Art, my body, my mind, and my life have changed dramatically. I have become stronger and more flexible; I am quicker, more agile (both physically and mentally); my concentration and focus have improved dramatically; I have seen my patience increase drastically. I am so much more concen-

COMMENTS
OF SOME
STUDENTS
. . .

197

trated on and dedicated to everything and everyone around me than I ever was before. In short, I have found a wellspring of positive energy in this Art.

Before I began taking these classes, I had tried this and that physical activity with enthusiasm but they failed to captivate me and keep me long in them. I always left out of boredom. This Art has been different for me—I have found it easy to dedicate myself to learning and attempting to perfect its movements because the challenges involved are mental as well as physical. I remember how hard some of the coordinations were for me in the beginning, and it still amazes me that I have come to understand and execute them almost effortlessly, yet still with speed and precision.

I cannot recommend this Art enough, for all of the changes that I have seen in myself, as well as in the others whom I have seen study it. It is challenging, positive, and a lot of fun.

Benjamin Kelley, twenty-five years old
teacher and tutor
United States

I have been taking these classes for the past seven months and I have seen a huge change in my body. I am physically much stronger and have increased my stamina and endurance level. Movements that were at first very difficult for me, both for strength and coordination, now feel more effortless, as though they have become a natural part of my being. While I am doing the movements, I am focused and clear. I have found that I can access that clarity very quickly when I start my practice. One thing that has surprised me is that I don't feel sore after class even though the movements are quite rigorous.

I have enjoyed challenging my body and maintaining the self-discipline to come to each class, even though the classes are early in the morning. I have recently passed the first stage and am eager and excited to learn new movements of the second stage that are based upon and at the same time different than what I have already learned.

In addition to the classes being a physical challenge, they have also had an impact on me mentally and emotionally. What I have noticed the most is that I want to do the movements correctly, and this desire in and of itself inhibits free, quick, and spontaneous movement. I have gotten coaching on letting go of doing it right and just being in my body and moving without thinking. I am very appreciative of that.

> Sara Bursac, twenty-four years old
> youth worker and yoga instructor
> United States

WHEN I started to study this Art over nine months ago, I was not sure that I would or could continue. I was barely able to complete the simplest movements. My goals at that time were increased flexibility, improved coordination and concentration, as well as relief from pain. I was in near constant pain from my feet. These classes have had a dramatic influence upon me. I have achieved all of my goals and then some!

I have gone from needing 12 to 16 ibuprofen per day to needing only 3 to 6 to relieve the pain in my feet.

My golf game has improved considerably as a result of my improved flexibilty and concentration.

I am able to walk one to two miles without any discomfort, an impossibility before.

My outlook on life has transformed from looking for the negative to looking for the positive in all situations.

When I think back to my first few lessons I am amazed at my progress; going from being unable to maintain my balance during most movements to completing and mastering a whole cycle of them.

I have recommended these classes to friends and coworkers and would encourage anyone to practice this Art.

> Richard G. Kelley, fifty-nine years old
> software developer and consultant
> United States

BASICALLY, this Art is not exercise for the lazy—but it has a magical effect on someone like me, who never sticks with any exercise program: it gives me an active connection between my mind and body, constant improvement, and a program I stick with because it's always new. While at first I was confused by its combination of (literally) jumpy activity and funny little exercises like eye motions, I soon learned that's how it kept my attention.

It's exercise that doesn't require you to have bulging muscles, feet that can go behind your head, or six-pack abs. Nor does it ask

you to behave like a monk or an athlete. Like any program it requires commitment, but gives you plenty of incentives to keep
coming (constant progress; just enough formality to give it a
"group effort" feel). It requires attention to really get anything out
of it, but it rewards that attention with challenges you can meet.

Michael T. Bullock, twenty-eight years old
musician and teacher
United States

In God Almighty's name, I truly and sincerely testify to the healing and restitution of my sick organs from a disease called "dis-
abling rheumatoid arthritis" that can be acquired by both young
and old. Now I am healthy thanks to the Seamm-Jasani classes
and the patience and dedication of my teacher.

I am delighted and truly thankful with my whole heart, since
with this Art I feel happy, young, beautiful, healthy, and glad to be
alive.

I love you from all my heart.

Elvia Cereceda, fifty-five years old
cosmetologist
Chile

We are writing this letter to let you know about our experiences
studying the Seamm-Jasani. We have seen so many good things
come from this Art, from gradual weight loss to better muscle
strength and tone to an achievement of physical harmony.

All of these have led to a better state of mind, which shows itself in our daily lives as well as in our relationships, showing us truly that a healthy body leads to a healthy mind.

The purpose of these few words is to express our deep gratitude toward you, our teacher, for how much we have progressed, both physically and mentally. We are looking forward to continuing this learning process, studying this Art that you teach so well.

Hoping these words express some of our feelings, and wishing you our best.

> Viviana Castillo, artisan
> Diana Sapaj, housewife
> Luis Araya, student

THESE techniques work from the deepest levels of our consciousness as we use movements and breathing to achieve a balance between our body and mind, and throughout our entire organism.

Its benefits are many, felt from the very first classes and in basic aspects of the student's personality: body, mind, emotions, volition.

This Art works to develop our entire organism, and in students one can observe an increase in individual productivity as the student begins to center on him or herself, beginning to understand the notion of synergy between body and mind.

> Leni Bossa
> clinical and business psychologist, lawyer
> Brazil

LEARNING these ancient teachings has shown me, both in my personal experience and from what I have seen in other students, that it is never too late to stop time and go back to the strength, vigor, and joy of youth.

> Jessica Martinez
> cosmetologist, physical therapist
> Argentina

THIS Art, as a discipline and from an athletic point of view, fulfills all of the standards, requirements, and objectives sought by physical education; that is to say that it is a practice that fully develops a person, both physically and mentally.

It can be practiced by anyone, without restrictions of age or gender, and can be used as rehabilitation and physical therapy. It develops motor skills that spread from our neurosensory perception to a wider spatial/temporal field through simple and complicated coordinative movements. It also improves our athleticism, along with strengthening our volition and mental prowess, leading us to a state of general health as it promotes and optimizes the general functioning of our organism, improving our respiratory, nervous, circulatory, and muscular systems. Mainly based in isotonic and isometric movements accompanied by opened and corrected breathing, it is a very effective discipline for enlarging our aerobic capacity while simultaneously enhancing us anaerobically.

Through constant and systematic training the student gains better muscle tone, corrects his or her posture, and comes to a balanced body weight. On the functional side of things, I have to say that physical abilities are also enhanced, improving strength, agility, speed, resistance, power, flexibility, and general ease of movement.

The movements executed by the students are completely natural and do not require any additional load as the only resistance is given by their own body as they move it in every direction, allowing for a physical development that is strictly individual, tailored to the needs of each student.

Felipe Cerna V.
physical education, sports, and recreation teacher
rugby national champion
rowing national champion,
single scull boats, double pair
Chile

In these agitated days of the twenty-first century, in which it is necessary to create time to spend with yourself, we can count on this theraputic tool, Seamm-Jasani, which lets us stop for a moment to recover strength and harmony in order to be able to progress through our lives with less stress. The key is not to hide from the world looking for self-improvement, since it is inside every one of us, inserted in each community. The Seamm-Jasani is a way to find that.

Fernando Bórquez R., MD
surgeon
Chile

SINCE beginning these classes, my life has changed in every way: my mood has improved and I feel younger, find myself full of vitality and energy, and do things that I really could not do before . . . I have not only found the source of youth, but also of positivity.

Marilyn Revello, forty-five years old
accountant

THESE relaxation and breathing exercises have been fantastic! I have been able to strengthen my spine, which had begun to bend, and the breathing exercises that we do have helped me relax, turning tense moments into ones of confidence. The movements themselves have helped me improve my memory, which had been affected by my age.

But what has been most important is that my concentration has improved. That is why I think so highly of this Art, because it has really helped me to develop myself.

Oscar Rogat, fifty-eight years old
businessperson

THESE classes have really helped out my nerves, especially my arthritic pains, and have helped me to sleep better than before. I am very happy with the whole course, because it is very useful and it makes me feel good.

Otilia Espinoza, seventy years old
housewife

My whole attitude, my state of mind, even how I rest, have all improved so much. I don't get so tired anymore and the classes really help me stay excited about things.

Olivia Cerpa, fifty-four years old
businessperson

My sincerest congratulations, because this beautiful discipline fills us with satisfaction and joy, because it is good for the body and for the spirit. In these classes I've found the energy I've needed, the companionship and the good feelings that make you wait impatiently for the next class. Everything about them is positive. I hope I can continue them for a long time.

Daniela Gonzalez, forty-eight years old
businessperson

I am so happy and grateful for these classes. When practicing this Art, I feel joy and I feel comfortable with my body. Being able to take these classes is such a great opportunity, because it takes me out of my routine so I forget my problems. It also helps my body clean itself out. Thanks to the people that teach us.

Regina Del Pino, forty-one years old
artisan

COMMENTS
OF SOME
STUDENTS
· · ·

I want to express my satisfaction with this course for active relaxation. From the very first classes I have seen the changes. I have learned how to breathe to purify my lungs, to be more coordinated, to keep myself balanced. That is why I say that this is an excellent discipline. Plus, it helps you stay calm.

Betty Cea, seventy years old
housewife

THROUGH studying this Art, I have found what I have always searched for: harmony with my body, internal tranquility, and energy—lots of positive energy that I can apply to achieving my goals.

It has given me the confidence and inner strength to develop myself in other areas of my life and to make myself into a more complete individual.

Why didn't I start before?

Jorge Henríquez R, forty-seven years old
architect

Further Information

Mmulargan: *School for the Boabom Arts*

Asanaro, author of this book and teacher of the arts described within, supervises and teaches at the Mmulargan School, a center for the Boabom Arts. These arts are grounded in the understanding that body and mind form a perfect unity, essential and complete. Within the Mmulargan School, three basic arts are taught:

✳   Seamm-Jasani, or the Art for Eternal Youth through fluid movements and meditation.

✳   Traditional Boabom, or the Art of Defense of the Inner Path, developed as a system of self-medicine, relaxation, and self-defense.

. . .

★   Yaan-Bao, or the Art of Elements. This system of move-ments, defense, and relaxation utilizes elements (such as staffs of various shapes and sizes) as extensions of the body.

For further information about the Mmulargan School, visit:

www.boabom.org

A branch of the Mmulargan School has recently opened in Boston, and there are plans to open similar schools in other loca-tions. For more information regarding these schools and the classes they offer, please contact:

Benjamin Kelley
boabomusa@hotmail.com

If you wish to contact the author or ask any questions regard-ing this book, please write to him!

asanaro58@yahoo.com

About the Author

Asanaro has dedicated more than twenty years to the study and teaching of Alternative Arts and Philosophy originating in pre-Buddhist Tibet, transmitted as thirty-three diverse sciences of relaxation, defense, meditation, and philosophy. Asanaro has taught around the world, offering courses and developing schools in South America, Europe, and the United States. He has also been instrumental in the founding and creation of many different centers and associations for alternative arts and medicine, including *Samsara,* a Chilean not-for-profit organization dedicated to alternative medicine and self-healing. He is the author of *Bamso: The Art of Dreams,* a guide to meditation and astral projection. He currently resides in Chile.